KU-677-753

MENDING THE BROKEN HEART

A Psychological Perspective on Preventing and Treating Heart Disease

by
Herbert S. Strean

1527666

LIBRARY

ACC. No. | DEPT.
0179816 | WITHDRAWN
CLASS No.
616.120019 STR

UNIVERSITY
COLLEGE CHESTER

JASON ARONSON INC.
Northvale, New Jersey
London

Director of Editorial Production: Robert D. Hack

This book was set in 12 pt. Times New Roman by ergo of Clifton, New Jersey, and printed by Book-mart Press of North Bergen, New Jersey.

Copyright © 1996 by Jason Aronson Inc.

10 9 8 7 6 5 4 3 2 1

All rights reserved. Printed in the United States of America. No part of this book may be used or reproduced in any manner whatsoever without written permission from Jason Aronson Inc. except in the case of brief quotations in reviews for inclusion in a magazine, newspaper, or broadcast.

Library of Congress Cataloging-in-Publication Data

Strean, Herbert S.
 Mending the broken heart : a psychological perspective on preventing and treating heart disease / Herbert S. Strean.
  p. cm.
 Includes bibliographical references and index.
 ISBN 0-7657-0010-7 (sc : alk. paper)
 1. Heart–Diseases–Psychological aspects. 2. Heart–Diseases--Psychosomatic aspects. I. Title.
RC682.S79 1997
616.1'2'0019–dc20   96-14383

Manufactured in the United States of America. Jason Aronson Inc. offers books and cassettes. For information and catalog write to Jason Aronson Inc., 230 Livingston Street, Northvale, New Jersey 07647.

This book is affectionately dedicated to my friends from Group 3C of the Dr. Dean Ornish Program at Beth Israel Hospital Medical Center, New York

To our leader, Lou Shankman, who always shows lots of heart, and to the members of Group 3C, who are always learning to do so:

Lee Aks
Cary Bell
Dan Blechman
Jerry Davidson
Bob Finkin
Arthur Fried
Mel Hartman
Gil Kiefer
Bernie Messina (in memoriam)
Henry Ostberg
Shelly Stachel
Anthony Surban (Assistant Leader)
Harold Weinberger
Tom Winter

"Ask not what disease the person has,
but rather what person the disease has."

An Anthropologist of Mars:
Some Paradoxical Tales
Oliver Sacks, M.D.

Table of Contents

Heart to Heart:
a Personal Prologue

It was Friday morning, April 1, 1994. I awoke feeling very sluggish and mildly depressed. As I reflected on my downcast mood, I realized I was preoccupied with many issues. That evening I was going to chair my last board meeting at the New York Center for Psychoanalytic Training. I had been the director of the Center for eight years and I had very mixed feelings about saying goodbye to my colleagues and friends. I found myself ruminating about all the tasks I had not accomplished, as well as those I had not performed too well.

While driving to my office, I felt a wave of sadness, and recalled that it was exactly one year to the day that the founder of the Center, my predecessor, mentor, and personal analyst, Dr. Reuben Fine, had passed away. For about three years prior to his death, he had been very ill, physically and emotionally. Consequently it had been very difficult for most of us who were close to him to relate to him in our usual warm and spontaneous manner. As I approached my office, I was speaking out loud in my car to Reuben as if he were alive and was a passenger: "Damn you! Instead of coming to the board meeting and expressing your good wishes, you are dead! And, instead of remembering you encouraging and supporting me the last couple of years, I recall all of the times you made it difficult for me. Right now I feel you are like a mean father."

As I heard myself say "mean father," I thought of my own father. After briefly recalling times he had been mean to me, with a startle it suddenly occurred to me that I had just turned 63 years old, an ominous age when I realized my father had died at 62. With some guilt, I told myself, "A son shouldn't be older than his father."

By the time I saw my first patient in psychotherapy, I was feeling quite agitated. In contrast to my usual posture with patients, which is one of warm concentration and relatedness, my mind was wandering and I kept watching the clock. It definitely was not my day!

As the day that was not mine went on, I felt increasingly tired and lonely. Inasmuch as this was not my usual state of mind, I knew something was going on in my unconscious that was deeply troubling. I said to myself, "Instead of listening to my patients and supervisees, I'd like to talk to somebody about me. Maybe to Reuben?"

Prior to the evening's board meeting, I ate a big dinner, which (I realized in the future) was full of fat—French fried potatoes, fried onion rings, and some other foods which were not particularly healthy, especially for an agitated fellow. Yet, I was partially aware that I was attempting to minister to my distress and loneliness.

Within 10 minutes after I called the board meeting to

order, I began feeling sensations which I had never felt in my 63 years of living. I was sweating profusely, my arms felt as if they were vibrating, and I had pressure in my chest. I tried my best to ignore the pains and aches, and in characteristic fashion attempted to conduct the meeting with grace and determination. It was difficult, but I persisted.

The sensations that I experienced at the beginning of the board meeting continued through the end of it 2 hours later. At times the pains were less severe. I was very relieved when I could finally say, "The meeting is adjourned." With tears in my eyes and my voice choking, I said to my colleagues, "This will be the last time I say that."

When I arrived home about 11:00 P.M. on the night of April lst, 1994, my wife, Marcia, took one look at me and immediately knew something was wrong. When I told her about my symptoms, she said, "Let's go to the hospital, those are heart attack symptoms." But I insisted it was indigestion and that I would be fine.

But, I was not fine. I didn't sleep well and was very tired the next day, Saturday, feeling chest and arm pains. At no point did I relate those pains to anything cardiovascular. I thought of a possible gall bladder problem, a "nervous stomach," and other maladies, even though there had been quite a bit of heart disease in my family—my two grandfathers died from heart attacks in their fifties and sixties, as did my father. But, I was different. Or, so I thought! On Sunday morning, April 3rd, the chest and arm pains grew worse. As I was experiencing much discomfort, I suddenly felt as if somebody was squeezing my chest and trying to sap my energy. That lasted about ten minutes, but I was still denying this was a heart attack.

My wife quickly arranged to take me to a local hospital.

Within moments, I was lying on a bed in the emergency room with tests being done. When enzymes were found in my blood and the emergency room doctor had ascertained from me that I had not had any recent injury, he told me firmly and sternly, "You have to be admitted to the hospital. It's the Intensive Care Unit for you. You've had a heart attack and you may have another one!"

The doctor's admonishing statements were the first of many physicians' remarks to me that were irritating and devasting to me! I asked myself, "No warmth, no sensitivity, no empathy? Just cold and mechanical directions? Is this supposed to help me?" As more physicians gave me more discouraging words such as, "You need to take at least six weeks off. You've had an attack," I became more agitated, more despondent, and had more fantasies about meeting my maker quite soon. I keenly felt what Norman Cousins (1983) wrote about in *The Healing Heart*, which was the indignity of the hospital environment, its mechanical atmosphere, and the inability of those charged with caring for heart patients to communicate constructively with them. I would read later in the books and articles by cardiologists and others who view the human being's feelings as more crucial to his recovery than anything else (for example, Benson 1976, Cannon 1963, Lazare 1987, Ornish 1990, Sacks 1995, Schneider 1967) that physicians do not learn in medical school how to communicate and that frequently their terse diagnostic statements, prescriptions, and proscriptions can induce panic. Of perhaps more importance, I learned later that panic exacerbates heart disease, and, as a result, many physicians with their callous remarks can induce heart problems rather than relieve them (Cousins 1976).

By the second day of my hospitalization, I was feeling

very frightened, weakened, and pessimistic. Intuitively, I knew this emotional state was not good for my heart condition. I was to read a few months later in a book by an eminent cardiologist, Bruno Cortis (1995), the following: "Feeling powerless, feeling afraid, and feeling that you are in the dark about what is going on are actually bad for the heart" (p. xviii).

The four days in the hospital seemed like an eternity. No reassuring remarks from anybody on the hospital staff seemed to be forthcoming, and I had no idea what my future would be. On the fourth day of my hospitalization, I was switched to another hospital to have an angiogram. Being on a stretcher in an ambulance made me feel like a weak cripple and I resented the idea that no one had prepared me for what was going to take place.

The next day, after I was in a dark room for about 45 minutes for the angiogram, the silent and detached physician uttered some very welcome words. He stated calmly, "You can be helped with medication. You do not need surgery." I was gleeful and thanked him profusely for his "kind remarks." Later, he drew me a diagram showing me that although I had one artery closed and another one operating at a 30 percent capacity, I had "a good collateral system." I was discharged from the hospital that night.

Other than prescriptions for medicines and a suggestion that I should exercise a lot after I "rest at home for awhile," I was given no instructions on how to conduct my life. I stayed home for a month, watched my diet carefully based on knowledge that my wife had, and slowly began to exercise. I was pleased that I did not need surgery and was grateful to be alive.

My relaxed attitude did not last too long. About a month

after I was discharged from the hospital, I was advised to take a stress test. I had never been on a treadmill in my life, and I was apprehensive about using one. I was also leery about what the test would yield.

Feeling much anxiety, I got on the treadmill at the office of a cardiologist new to me. My gait was wobbly and I was uncertain about how to perform. The doctor shouted direction after direction at me, and I became angrier and angrier, more and more breathless, and was feeling very vulnerable and awkward. Within 2 minutes he stopped the treadmill, saying, "You need bypass surgery immediately. You have *two* closed arteries and another one almost closed. You are functioning as if you are 85 years old!" He looked white with anxiety himself.

I wanted to hit the doctor in the jaw but left his office saying I would think over his advice. I think my body language showed him I did not welcome his remarks. As if to deny the severity of the doctor's ominous proclamations, I went that afternoon to a golf driving range and swatted some golf balls. I recall telling myself that the treadmill was a "dreadmill."

As I reflected more on my experiences with cardiologists and their associates, their lack of emotional sensitivity, their contradictions of each other, and the resentment they induced in me, I felt I had to take my future into my own hands. I needed help from those who seemed more positively responsive to me.

During the next several months I read dozens of books and articles on the treatment and prevention of heart disease. I became particularly impressed with the work of Dr. Dean Ornish, whose book my children gave me for Father's Day. He compassionately described his program of cardiac rehabilitation. This program prescribed a life style change involving daily exercise, daily stress reduction procedures, a fat-free vegetarian diet, and group support.

Rejecting the idea of bypass surgery, I entered Dr. Ornish's program in New York City at the Beth Israel Hospital in August 1994. Still actively involved in the program, my health has improved enormously, and my life and mood have changed dramatically. I often feel like a college student, full of vigor and optimism.

As I have shared my experiences with dozens of patients who have had heart disease, interviewed many cardiac patients at Beth Israel hospital and elsewhere, and asked my colleagues to refer psychotherapy patients with heart problems, I have arrived at some important convictions about the treatment and prevention of heart problems. These convictions, emanating from the extensive reading, research, and participant observation I have done, have been translated into this book.

My first and foremost conviction is that although daily exercise, stress reduction practices, and a healthy diet are important ingredients in the treatment and prevention of heart disease, coping with emotions, mastering anxiety, and resolving emotional conflicts are equally as important, if not more so. A corollary of this proposition is that although genetics, diet, and so forth are important variables to examine in assessing the etiology of heart disease, knowing about the individual's coping mechanisms, particularly how he or she deals with stressful situations and their attendant emotions is equally as crucial, if not more so.

As my own experience with physicians and hospital personnel attest, most of them do not experience their patients as unique individuals who have special strengths and vulnerabilities. Consequently, what has lagged in the growing body of knowledge on heart disease is the psychological understanding of the patient who suffers from heart disease or is likely to do so. This book is an attempt to enhance the psychological sophistication of professionals and nonprofessionals who want to know more about the person with heart problems, and to help him or her to resolve them.

Although not a new concept, my research into and personal experiences with heart disease have convinced me that the mind and body constantly interact, and that a healthy psyche can help make a healthy soma, and vice versa. Most modern cardiologists (for example, Benson 1976, Cortis 1995, Ornish 1990) subscribe to this point of view. This notion, according to Peter Gay (1988), one of Freud's major biographers, is probably one of Freud's most far reaching discoveries—that is, our unconscious minds and the thoughts, feelings, memories, and fantasies therein, are intimately connected with our bodily functions throughout our lives. In his recent book, *Heart and Soul*, Bruno Cortis (1995) avers: "It is becoming increasingly well known that the mind and body work together. The mind can affect the heart to the point of creating heart disease" (p.31).

Not only are the mind and body in constant transaction, but they are symbiotically linked—inseparable. Further, the brain (part of the mind) and the heart (part of the body) are in constant interaction so that emotions which are managed by the brain constantly influence the heart's activities, and the circulatory system always has an impact on the way we feel (Schneider 1967, Schur 1951). As Ornish (1990) has pointed out, considerable research has demonstrated that the brain produces certain molecules—neuropeptides—which interact with all of the cells of the body. Therefore, all emotional reactions produce neuropeptides, and each cell of the body is receptive to them. The emotions which first appear in the brain always end up influencing the body, particularly the heart.

Studying the mind–body transaction, particularly the close relationship between the brain and the heart, has led me to another important conviction, namely, that intense emotions which are not well-monitored, particularly those which cause stress, can and do lead to cardiac arrest, heart attacks, and other cardiovascular difficulties. One of the main reasons I have been very eager to write this book is to demonstrate how emotional conflicts which go unverbalized and unresolved are almost always in evidence when one assesses heart problems. I have felt that what I have learned in hindsight—that emotional conflicts and unmanaged, intense, emotional reactions are a major etiological factor in heart disease—can be utilized by others, but with foresight.

While being obsessively preoccupied with how the brain and emotions impact on the heart, I have been very impressed with the research of Meyer Friedman and Ray Rosenman (1981), who have demonstrated that a Type A Personality is more inclined to have heart disease than any of the other personality types. The Type A Personality, according to the authors, is an individual who is very ambitious, self-involved, always in a hurry, quite hostile, and cynical.

Participating in the Support Group in Dr. Dean Ornish's program at Beth Israel Hospital, interviewing heart patients, researching the literature, and constantly examining myself have led me to the conviction that virtually every man and woman who suffers from heart disease is a Type A personality.

However, Type A behavior tells us only a small part of the

heart disease story. Friedman and Rosenman's research deals primarily with symptoms of an unresearched personality. Why, for example, is the Type A individual hostile? What causes his or her intense ambitiousness? Why is he or she inclined to do many things, such as watch a basketball game, read the newspaper, and write a book—all at the same time?

The bulk of this book is an attempt to examine the Type A person in more breadth and depth and answer questions such as the ones above. My research has yielded the finding that propelling the ambitiousness of the Type A personality are intense omnipotent fantasies which are constantly clamoring for gratification. Because the individual under discussion can never attain the status of God, he or she is almost always angry. However, most of the time the anger is unacceptable to the individual, so he or she represses and suppresses it. Then the body is acutely affected and heart disease often results.

As I have intensively studied Type A behavior, I have noted not only the ubiquity of omnipotent fantasies and undischarged hostility but that problems of unresolved dependency, inhibitions in communication, and anxieties about loving and being intimate are also present. Observing how all of these characteristics—problems with omnipotence, dependency, hostility, communication, and so forth interact and transact, I have postulated the existence of "a cardiac personality," a person who is almost always under stress and usually experiences considerable loneliness.

As the chapters ahead will demonstrate, the *cardiac personality* also has many strengths. He or she usually has a good sense of humor, is intelligent, usually honest, law abiding, and loyal. The gregariousness of this person, however, is deceptive, because underneath his or her outgoing disposition is a very lonely individual. James Lynch (1985) in *The Language of the Heart: The Human Body in Dialogue* was the first to demonstrate that single, unattached individuals, who are often quite lonely, have a higher proportion of heart problems than do the rest of the population. Other researchers (for example, Cortis 1995, Ornish 1990) have formed similar conclusions.

As a dynamically oriented psychotherapist, my major professional interest and activity for the past 40 years has involved assessing people's dynamics and helping them to resolve their problems. Consequently, throughout this book, each chapter, with the exception of Chapter 1, will contain vignettes of real people who are suffering or have suffered from heart problems. (Names and other identifying data are disguised to protect confidentiality.) In the first part of each chapter (except Chapter 1), we will concern ourselves with the psychodynamics of our subjects, and in the second part of the chapter we will discuss therapeutic procedures that helped them resolve their emotional conflicts.

In Chapter 1, "The Heart That's Been Beaten," we will first discuss the frequency of heart disease in the 1990s and what is being done about it. We will demonstrate that in most instances the role of the emotions and emotional conflicts are very much neglected. We will then discuss the importance of viewing the mind and body as a gestalt in constant transaction and that overlooking this transactional gestalt neglects the heart patient diagnostically and therapeutically.

"Stressing the Heart," Chapter 2, will show how the concept of "stress" has been ambiguously defined. Although a crucial factor in the etiology and treatment of heart problems, stress needs to be more precisely defined. This is the main objective of Chapter 2. In Chapter 2 we will also try to show how stress is always linked to heart problems and its reduction is necessary if the heart patient is to function more adaptively.

In Chapter 3 we will present the cardiac personality as a complex individual who has many maladaptive character traits but many strengths. By being able to identify this person, mental health professionals and others will be in a much better position to help prevent heart disease and enhance its treatment. In this chapter we will also consider some of the major therapeutic principles that work with the cardiac personality.

Chapters 4 to 7 deal with major character traits of the cardiac personality. In these chapters we will examine the history, dynamics, values, vulnerabilities, defenses, and significant relationships of heart patients as well as the therapeutic attitudes that can be helpful to them in resolving their emotional conflicts.

In Chapter 4, "From Omnipotence to Competence," we will attempt to show why the cardiac personality is continually preoccupied with omnipotent fantasies and show that he or she can learn to tame them. In "From Rage to Healthy Assertion," Chapter 5, we will try to demonstrate why rage is an inevitable response when one is consistently egocentric and ambitious, and we will also elucidate how rage can be diminished.

One of the frequently unnoticed problems of cardiac personalities is their repressed yearning to be given to, but which they frequently deny. Through our case illustrations in Chapter 6, entitled "From Pseudo-independence to Healthy Dependency," we will try to show how unacceptable dependency wishes can be channelled into healthy attachment.

The cardiac personality frequently has a strict conscience (a punitive superego). Consequently, he or she judges himself or herself severely and does the same with others. In Chapter 7, "From Harsh Judgments to Constructive Communication," we will try to show how patients can be helped to conduct a healthier and more constructive dialogue with themselves and others.

In the final chapter, Chapter 8, "Love Is the Answer," we will attempt to show that by reducing hatred and increasing the capacity to love, the heart patient can become a healthier human being physically and mentally. The epilogue will summarize all of our findings and present our major conclusions.

No book is the sole product of the labors of one person. I would like to thank the many individuals who helped to make this book a reality.

First, to my wife, Marcia, who has been on my side through health and illness, good and bad times, my loving appreciation. In addition to her many complex roles, she has edited and typed drafts of this and many of my other books.

To my sons, Dr. Richard Strean and Dr. Billy Strean and to my daughter-in-law, Dr. Wendy Rodgers, who always keep me on my toes, asking good questions about the merits of psychotherapy and the limitations of psychotherapeutic research, my profound gratitude and love.

To all of the patients who entrusted their lives to me in psychotherapy and who furnished much of the data which are on the forthcoming pages, my gratitude for being such able consultants.

To the many patients at Beth Israel Medical Center, particularly those in Dr. Dean Ornish's program, my thanks for having opened my eyes and ears to sights and sounds I would never have seen or heard.

I would like to thank my colleagues at Jason Aronson Inc.

for helping this book become a reality. To Jason Aronson, M.D., and Michael Moskowitz, Ph.D., my gratitude for being receptive to my controversial ideas. To the Director of Author Relations, Norma Pomerantz, my thanks for promoting my books with good taste and tact. Finally, much appreciation goes to Bob Hack, Director of Editorial Production, for being an expert with all the nitty-gritty aspects of book production.

As the dedication page of this book shows, I am particularly indebted to my friends in Group 3C of the Ornish Program at Beth Israel, who, in addition to giving me much research data, have helped me to appreciate the beauty, wonder, and pleasure of warm friendship.

Finally, my profound gratitude to the able, sensitive, and empathetic staff of the Ornish Program at Beth Israel Medical Center, which is under the direction of Steven Horowitz, M.D. Many thanks to Shari Behar and Jane Kustin who taught us how to exercise. Much warmth to Laurie Jones who was always a charming and efficient program coordinator and, in addition, taught us how to eat right. Thanks to Elizabeth Kapstein, the chef who always gave us healthy and delicious food. Much appreciation goes to Deborah Matza and Luis Sierra, who taught us how to manage stress. Also many thanks to Roberto Roberti, M.D., physician coordinator, for his consistent medical attention. Finally, to two individuals who are now friends, group support leaders Louis Shankman and Charles Leighton, my abiding gratitude.

July 1, 1996
New York, NY

1

The Heart That's Been Beaten

Heart disease is America's Number One killer. Over forty million individuals in the United States suffer from diagnosed cardiovascular disease and an even larger number are not aware that they have heart problems. Sixty million people have high blood pressure. Eighty million people have high cholesterol levels. Each year over one-and-a-half million Americans have a heart attack, which means every twenty seconds someone in the United States is having a heart attack. One third of these heart attacks are fatal (Ornish 1990).

Although traditionally confined to men, heart disease is the leading killer of women, too. As the role-sets of women have become more complex, as the stresses in their lives increase, more women fall prey to heart disease. Slightly more than half the deaths from heart disease in the United States occur among women and this share is likely to increase as the population ages. One in 9 women aged 45 to 64 has some form of heart or blood vessel disease, and this ratio soars to

1 in 3 at age 65 and beyond. Furthermore, heart attacks or their aftermath tend to be more deadly in women. About one quarter more women than men die within a year of having a heart attack. (This difference may stem from women generally being older than men when they suffer heart attacks) (Patlak 1994). Recent comments include women not getting the same care as men.

Heart disease now accounts for more deaths than cancer and AIDS. The cost of cardiovascular disease in the United States is well over $125 billion dollars each year. Not only does heart disease affect both sexes, but now 156,000 Americans under the age of 65 die of this disease annually. Forty-five percent of all fatal heart attacks strike people under the age of 65, and 5 percent strike people under 40 (Cortis 1995).

Despite the fact that there is unanimous agreement on the incidence of heart disease, and although there is no lack of consensus about the severity of the problem, there is a great deal of controversy regarding the etiology, treatment, and prevention of heart disease.

What Is Heart Disease?

Facts and facsimiles

Virtually all cardiologists and other experts agree that when deposits of cholesterol grow on the inside of the arteries, the amount of blood that passes through is reduced and the heart gets less fuel. As the arteries get narrower, the heart suffers. The lack of blood and oxygen causes chest pains, technically referred to as *angina pectoris*. Cholesterol blockages can, abruptly, become covered by the formation of a blood clot, and the result is a complete occlusion of the artery. This causes a heart attack whereby chest pains grow in intensity and frequency and part of the heart eventually becomes damaged (Charash 1991, Cortis 1995, Ornish 1990, Schneider 1967).

Heart attacks are most likely to occur during the hours before or after dawn. One reason may be that platelets, which are stickiest then, may clump and form clots that can trigger heart attacks (*Consumer Reports on Health,* August 1991).

Cholesterol

Cholesterol is a national obsession (Charash 1991) with almost everyone talking about lowering his or her cholesterol level. Yet, few Americans know what cholesterol is, and fewer are aware of the many controversies surrounding the subject.

Cholesterol is a fatlike substance that is used by every cell in the body to form cell membranes. It is also utilized to create some hormones and other vital body chemicals. Cholesterol in the blood transports fats from the liver to the cells for storage. LDL and HDL cholesterol refer to the special molecules that transport cholesterol and fats through the blood. Low-density lipoproteins (LDL) carry cholesterol from the liver to the body tissues, while high-density lipoproteins (HDL) carry cholesterol from the arteries to the liver. If one has too many LDLs relative to HDLs, excess cholesterol tends to be deposited on the arterial walls, leading to arteriosclerosis. The HDL is often known as the good cholesterol because it can remove the bad LDL from the arterial walls and return it to the liver for excretion (Cortis 1995).

Although there is agreement among the experts that excessive cholesterol can be harmful because when it makes deposits in the walls of the arteries throughout the body to form plaque (hardening of the arteries or *atherosclerosis*) and thereby the risk of heart attacks increases, there is much disagreement about what a cholesterol level should be.

Many physicians aver that the risk of heart disease decreases when the cholesterol level is two hundred milligrams or less. Therefore, they conclude that it is very important to be aware of one's cholesterol level at all times. In 1992, *Consumer Reports on Health*, though recommending that one should always watch the cholesterol level, stated categorically that "most heart attacks occur in people whose cholesterol level is less than 240 mg/dl, the traditional cutoff for a dangerous score" (p. 59).

Bruce Charash (1991), author of *Heart Myths*, has pointed out that the idea of a normal cholesterol level is invalid and unreliable. Although acknowledging that the risk of heart disease is extremely high with a cholesterol level of 330 and is much lower with a level of under 180, "the risk is continuous [and] there is no absolutely safe level" (p. 5). Rather than looking for "a normal level," which is too difficult to define, Charash suggests that increments often should be viewed as increasing the risk of heart disease. In effect, he suggests that we dispense with the notion of "a normal level" and instead focus on "incremental acceleration."

Many individuals incorrectly believe that a low cholesterol level means they cannot have a heart attack. However, if the focus is placed on increments, many individuals will be receiving appropriate warning which they now lack.

When cholesterol was labelled as an enemy several

decades ago, most food manufacturers boasted about their cholesterol-free products. Yet, many individuals did not and do not realize that if they eat less cholesterol, the body makes more. Therefore, eating less cholesterol may not be the most effective way of reducing the risk of heart disease. Many authors (Charash 1991, Cortis 1995, Ornish 1990) recommend that the way to reduce heart disease is to abstain from foods that contain saturated fat and oil. Eating less fat and oil is what lessens the production of cholesterol, as does the abstinence from smoking. Nonetheless, there is ongoing debate about whether certain unsaturated fats and fish oils (such as in salmon) will reduce the production of cholesterol.

In sum, although the American Heart Association (1978) and other governmental agencies have taken the position that lowering the cholesterol intake always insures a longer life, the empirical facts do not justify this claim. [Recently in *The Menninger Letter* (April 1995) it was reported that a low cholesterol level can lead to depression and even thoughts of suicide.] Although there is much more to be examined about cholesterol, and despite the fact that much data now collected needs more validation, we can say and with some conviction that lessening the intake of saturated fat and oils and dispensing with smoking can reduce the possibility of heart disease.

Exercise

In addition to a fat-free diet, most experts who advocate ways and means of reducing heart disease recommend exercise. However, the quality and quantity of the exercise is still being debated. One day we learn in the media that only one type of exercise will reduce heart disease (for example,

Jane Brody, April 19, 1995, *New York Times,* "Only Vigorous Exercise Routine Adds Years to Life," p. l). Yet, the next day we will read that something else has been shown to be effective, negating what we learned the previous day. For example, in the Spring 1995 issue of *Good Medicine,* it was reported by Andrew Nicholson that patients suffering from heart disease were evaluated after five years of rehabilitation and those that participated in moderate exercise were doing the best.

While there has been an explosive public interest in exercising,with all kinds of benefits promised (including improving the memory function in the elderly and slowing the rate of age-related mental deterioration) (*The Menninger Letter,* April 1995), scientific studies performed to date have not convincingly demonstrated that exercising results in an improved survival rate. It can certainly improve the mood, lower the level of cholesterol, and have other positive effects such as muscular flexibility, but as yet it has not been demonstrated that exercise prolongs life. As Charash (1991) has stated:

> Physical training results in a sense of well-being because of other effects: 1. it improves the efficiency of the muscles of the arms and legs; 2. it improves the hormonal tone of the body, resulting in a lower blood pressure and heart rate; 3. it lowers the level of cholesterol and 4. it improves the control of sugar in people with diabetes. However, exercise will not make the heart beat more strongly. [p.223]

Despite the fact that some physicians proscribe exercise for individuals with heart problems, these doctors tend to be in the minority. It is now fairly well accepted that the risk of having a heart attack during exercise is small. Sudden cardiac death is very infrequent among athletes and when it does occur, abnormalities of the heart had been present for some time (Schneider 1967). In a study that examined men who joined an exercise program within 15 weeks of experiencing a heart attack, it was found that the heart muscle became weaker. However, it was concluded that the exercising was premature (Charash 1991).

An exercise test, often called "a stress test" also has its champions and detractors. The stress test is a means of observing the performance of the heart with an electrocardiogram during a period of gradually increasing levels of physical activity, usually on a treadmill. In an FDA Consumer Report, published in November 1994, it was concluded that the standard stress treadmill test falsely predicts heart disease in as many as half of those tested. However, other reports (e.g., *Consumer Reports on Health,* August 1992) report more reliable results.

Alcohol

Most nonprofessionals are familiar with the old and still ongoing debate regarding alcohol and its effects in the prevention and treatment of heart disease. The media frequently report studies that demonstrate that those who consume alcohol in mild amounts have slightly less heart disease than those who abstain. Yet many physicians (for example, Charash 1991) have noted that alcohol is toxic to all cells in the body, including the heart. Also, there is a heart condition known as alcoholic cardiomyopathy caused by the direct poisoning of the cells of the heart by alcohol. The symptoms are: severe weakness of the heart, body weakness, shortness of breath, and the death of 50 percent to 80 percent of its victims within three years.

Inasmuch as the responses to alcohol vary a great deal from person to person (and there may be some genetic predisposition which influences the response), perhaps some individuals' hearts are harmed by alcohol while other individuals may actually benefit somewhat from it.

Aspirin and Other Medications

As is true with most of the variables surrounding the treatment and prevention of heart disease, there is much ambivalence about the use of medications. Most patients who have had heart problems are given prescriptions for several types of medications immediately. Usually they are pleased to use them in order to help themselves. However, in a very short time, they are eager to get off their prescribed medications. Their ambivalence is often mirrored by their physicians.

All medications have their toxic and tonic effects. A good example is aspirin. It can lower temperature, relieve aches and inflammation, and can interfere with blood clotting. But it can also be responsible for bleeding problems and other side effects such as ringing in the ears, fatigue, stomach irritations, and ulcers. Hemorrhagic strokes and sudden cardiac death can also result. Further, aspirin does not affect coronary atherosclerosis; the blockages continue to build up over time (Ornish 1990).

Cardiologists and physicians in general, like all other human beings, have their idiosyncrasies and biases. Many of them champion medications of all types and believe that one who has heart disease should use medications indefinitely. Others, such as those in the Ornish program, are pleased and proud to announce when patients are *not* using cholesterol-lowering drugs and other medications.

It should not be overlooked in any review of the role of medications on heart disease that drugs are a big and booming business. Consequently, the patient's welfare is not always in the forefront. In *Deadly Medicine*, Moore (1995) has demonstrated how the successful promoting of the drug Tambocor caused cardiac arrests in hundreds of patients.

Bypass Surgery

One of the most popular forms of treatment for heart disease is bypass surgery. Many cardiologists recommend this procedure after a patient has suffered a heart attack, particularly if an angiogram or stress test reveal clogged arteries. More often than not, the physicians are trying to protect themselves, as much if not more than they want to help the patient, concerned that if the patient has another heart attack, the doctor will be held responsible. Bypass surgery is currently the most common major operation performed in the United States; more than 250,000 are performed each year (Charash 1991).

In a coronary bypass, a section of a clean vein (often from the leg) is inserted to detour blood flow around the diseased artery. Designed to avoid blockages and restore normal blood flow to the heart, the goals of bypass surgery are to relieve chest pains and prevent heart attacks.

As popular as bypass surgery is, several authors have

focused on several of its limitations. Cortis (1995) says: "As for a coronary bypass, the procedure literally bypasses the problem.... The cause of the heart disease, the reasons for the artery being clogged, remains and can recur" (p. 5).

Ornish (1990) notes: "In the early 1980s, three major randomized, controlled clinical studies were published demonstrating that bypass surgery provided only marginal benefit for most patients with moderate to severe heart disease... In other words, many of the patients who underwent bypass surgery didn't really need it" (p. 52). Dr. Ornish also remarks:

> New problems occur (heart attacks, strokes, infection, or death can occur during the bypass surgery, and up to one third of patients who undergo bypass surgery suffer some transient or permanent neurological damage or decrease in I.Q.), the old problem may recur or persist (fifty percent of bypassed arteries clog up again within five years, and eighty percent become blocked after seven years). Similarly,...the incidence of strokes was higher in people who underwent bypass surgery. [pp. 52-53]

Charash (1991) has concluded that bypass surgery has several limitations:

1. Damaged heart muscle will remain damaged. A bypass operation has little, if any, effect on heart muscle strength.
2. Some of the narrowed arteries cannot be fixed by bypass surgery.
3. Blockages continue to develop and grow in the arteries of the heart during the years after a bypass

operation.

4. The bypass grafts can totally shut down, resulting in complete blockage.

5. The bypass surgery does not prevent future heart attacks.

6. The surgery can be fatal.

In sum, bypass surgery can prolong life in selected groups of heart patients. It does not prevent heart attacks but frequently can be effective in relieving symptoms of angina. The surgery cannot be considered a permanent solution.

Balloon Angioplasty

In 1977, Dr. Andreas Gruentzig invented balloon angioplasty. It is considered a much less invasive approach than bypass surgery. In this procedure, a balloon is passed through a tube inside a blocked artery. The balloon is inflated, squishing the blockage and making more room for blood to flow.

As Ornish (1990) has pointed out, because it was less traumatic for patients, angioplasty also gave cardiologists a tool to recapture from cardiac surgeons much of their lost status and income. In 5 years, the number of angioplasties went from 32,000 in 1983 to about 200,000 in 1988.

As is true with most interventive procedures in treating heart disease, angioplasty has its disadvantages and limitations. Sometimes arteries dissect or rupture when the balloon is inflated, thus requiring emergency bypass surgery. One third of arteries dilated by angioplasty will close up again within 4 to 6 months. Although designed to prevent heart attacks, angioplasty sometimes causes them. In the first 3,000 cases, close to 5 percent of the patients had a heart attack during angioplasty, and close to 9 percent required emergency bypass surgery (Ornish 1990).

Similar to bypass surgery, angioplasty does not insure the patient that it will be effective forever. Usually within 6 months, up to 30 percent of all arteries that are repaired will renarrow (called *restenors*) and this requires a second or third effort. Although bypass surgery has been demonstrated to improve survival in selected patients, it is not known whether this applies for balloon angioplasty. As Charash (1991) concludes: "Angioplasty is not known to offer an improvement in long-term health" (p. 85).

High Blood Pressure

As we mentioned at the beginning of this chapter, as many as 60 million Americans have high blood pressure, but many of them (35 percent) do not know they have it. High blood pressure, or hypertension, injures the coronary artery lining and leads to the formation of coronary blockages. When blood pressure rises, the blood hits the arterial wall forcibly, thereby causing injury to the lining of the artery. As the pressure increases, more injury to the lining of the arteries occurs, causing more blockages. Most experts agree (Charash 1991, Cortis 1995, Ornish 1990) that high blood pressure increases the risk of coronary heart disease.

The majority of physicians treat high blood pressure by prescribing antihypertensive drugs. According to the statistics of the American Heart Association, over 25 million Americans are taking antihypertensive drugs. These drugs for the most part are effective in lowering blood pressure in most people. However, as the reader can now anticipate, the side effects of antihypertensive drugs can be many: impotence, fatigue, depression, and blood cell disorders. Furthermore, many studies (Cutler et al. 1989, Kaplan 1987, Langford 1989) have demonstrated that decreasing blood pressure with drugs does not significantly reduce coronary heart disease mortality. As Ornish (1990) discovered, in approximately half of the studies examining the effect of drug treatment on hypertension, nonintervention control groups had fewer nonfatal heart attacks and fewer fatal heart attacks than the group treated with drugs.

Benson (1976,1977) and Ornish (1990) have independently learned that patients' blood pressure remains significantly reduced after making lifestyle changes that include a fat-free diet, exercise, stress reduction, meditation, and group support.

Treating and Preventing Heart Disease: A Subjective Approach?

As was indicated in the prologue, when I asked three different physicians how long I should spend resting and recovering from my heart attack, I received three different answers. The cardiologist in charge of my treatment told me gravely that I needed at least 6 weeks away from work because I had a "real heart attack." Another cardiologist recommended 4 weeks because I had "a minor attack" and my own internist told me that 2 weeks would be adequate because I was "eager to get back to work."

During the month I was recuperating, I wanted to go on a short vacation (about 3 to 4 days) which my wife and I had planned for some time. Again I solicited advice from three different physicians and again I got three different answers. One told me without any hesitation that I definitely should not go away. Another told me that I could be the judge. And the third said, "Feel free to go."

When I noted that different physicians had different responses to the idea of a brief trip for me, I began to do a little informal research. I asked the cardiologist who told me I could go away what the basis was for his advice. "You're going to Tennessee. I'd never miss that if I had the opportunity."

In response to my interest regarding his motives, the physician who told me I shouldn't go replied, "To be on the safe side, I always tell my patients not to travel for at least a month." (I wasn't able to do any "research" with the physician who told me that I could be the judge.)

The lack of agreement between three trained and experienced physicians regarding my rest and recuperation, I have learned, is par for the course. Hundreds of cardiac patients have reported similar experiences and many writers (for example, Cousins 1976, 1983) have noted that prescriptions, proscriptions, and treatment plans of physicians vary considerably.

As we have been noting throughout this chapter, those in charge of the treatment and prevention of heart disease often divide into camps, similar to feuding religious sects or political parties. Bypass surgery has its opponents and proponents as does angioplasty and the use of medications. How to exercise and how to read a cholesterol count continue to be debated. Physicians cannot agree whether alcohol is good or bad for heart disease. Although programs that prescribe a combination of a non-fat vegetarian diet, exercise, stress reduction, and group support have yielded empirical data showing numerous benefits (for example, Benson 1977, Chopra 1993, Ornish 1990), many cardiologists regard these programs as fads that are unreliable and invalid. Whether genetic endowment is a major etiological determinant in heart disease is still being argued. Although we know that heart disease tends to run in families, many writers point out that this does not affirm a genetic causation. It could be that stressful family atmospheres can be duplicated over the generations (Freedman et al. 1976).

In many ways the problems in diagnosing and treating heart disease are similar to those in diagnosing and treating schizophrenia. Just as there are those who contend that schizophrenia is an inherited biological disease and will argue vehemently with those who view schizophrenia as the outcome of conflicted interpersonal experiences, the same situation exists regarding heart disease, wherein the pure biologists strongly oppose other perspectives. Further, just as there are those treating schizophrenia who insist on treating the disease through drugs and concomitantly demean psychotherapy, there are many heart specialists who have a narrow focus and seriously question practices such as meditation, stress reduction, and group support.

For those of us in the mental health field, the subjectivity in the diagnosis, treatment, and prevention of heart disease comes as no surprise. Most psychotherapists recognize that a clinical diagnosis, a treatment plan, and a therapeutic intervention in psychotherapy cannot be assessed unless we know something about the psychodynamics of the clinician (Fine 1982, Strean 1993a). In fact, if one takes even a superficial glimpse at the life stories of some of the leading theorists in psychotherapy, the basis of his or her major tenets become quite clear. To make my point, though a digression from heart disease per se, I include the next paragraph.

Alfred Adler, who contended that the actions of human beings are essentially motivated by what they deem is "inferior" about themselves, was a small, sickly boy who felt dominated by another brother (Adler 1967). Karen Horney was the daughter of a sea captain who abandoned her frequently to go on voyages. She took the position that neuroses are caused by a feeling of "loneliness in a hostile world" (Kelman and Vollmerhausen 1967). Harry Stack Sullivan spent much of his childhood by himself alone on a farm. He founded the interpersonal school of psychiatry and took the position that every child, to grow to full maturity, needs a chum (Perry 1982). And, Sigmund Freud, who postulated the oedipus complex, slept in the parental bedroom for many years (Jones 1953).

Perhaps physicians, like psychotherapists, can learn as part of their training that their own childhood experiences, personal idiosyncracies, biases, fantasies, fears, and so forth strongly influence their medical evaluations, treatment plans, and interventions. As they do so, perhaps they can relate to the patients on a more individualized basis, controlling and eventually mastering their own prejudices and other subjective inclinations. As they see themselves more as total persons, they may be more enabled to see their patients as total people.

One of the serious weaknesses in medical practice is the failure to appreciate consistently that a patient's stresses, in the past and the present, contribute in a major way to the patient's current disease. Although it is now well documented that stress is an important factor in the etiology and continuation of heart disease, with many studies demonstrating convincing results (Alexander 1939, Arlow 1952, Ax 1953, Grollman 1929, Lacey and Van Lehn 1952, Reiser et al. 1955, Schacter 1957) these crucial findings are not being sufficiently utilized by the majority of physicians in their treatment and preventive work with heart disease.

The strong psychological component of heart disease—which the pages ahead will expose—has been neglected in work with heart patients. How is the patient experiencing his or her marriage, children, work? What neurotic conflicts have influenced the development of his or her heart problems? What psychological problems have been induced because of the patient's heart disease? How does the patient feel toward the doctor and how does the doctor feel toward the patient? How does the patient experience emotionally the doctor's interventions? These questions and others are always pertinent in work with the heart patient and need to be addressed.

The Contribution of the Psychotherapist

Although most psychotherapists are very willing to take stock of themselves as they try to help their patients, their continued emphasis on self-awareness has not helped them much in working with patients who have heart disease (and/or other physical maladies). Despite the fact that mental health workers can appreciate the notion that emotional problems contribute to bodily ills, like physicians who neglect their patients' psyches, most psychotherapists neglect their patients' somas.

Nine out of ten therapists, if presented with a patient who has a heart problem, will refer the patient to a physician and *not work* with the medical specialist on the mind–body problem before them. This sharp division of labor can only place limitations on the patient's possibility of recovering.

Inasmuch as it is the thesis of this book that heart disease is a mind-body problem, it is my strong conviction that its treatment requires the integrated thinking and activity of the physician and the psychotherapist. If the physician discovers that a patient is suffering from heart disease and/or has had a heart attack, the physician and the patient should be able to consult with a therapist so that the latter can determine the stresses in the patient's life and help the patient resolve them. Similarly, as psychotherapists learn to identify the cardiac personality with more precision, they will be better able to refer the patient to a cardiologist or other physician for the medical attention the patient needs.

Physicians and psychotherapists both need to know how and why the patient's stressful life has helped create his or her heart problem and both need to know how and why the heart problem creates stress. Psychotherapist and physician need to know how to complement and supplement their respective interventions while working with the whole person, whether the whole person has had a heart ailment or has tendencies in that direction.

Thus, based on my experiences as a heart patient, psychotherapist, and researcher, it is my strong conviction that heart disease is a mind–body problem, that is, a psychosomatic disease. In the remaining sections of this chapter, I wish to review some of the major issues that are important to those of us who utilize a mind–body perspective. This should make the following chapters on stress, the cardiac personality and his or her conflicts more comprehensible to those who wish to help patients reverse their heart disease.

The Mind–Body Perspective

In 1982 a study by three cardiologists, Kaplan, Manuck, and Clarkson, provided "the best scientific evidence to date of the role of emotional stress in causing coronary artery blockages" (Ornish 1990, p. 77). Kaplan and his collaborators experimented with cynomolgus monkeys (who are very similar to people in how they develop artery blockages).

Cynomolgus monkeys have a complex social organization and are keenly aware of their social rankings. The experimenters were able to determine the monkey's social rankings by reviewing the outcomes of competitive fights among the monkeys; winners of fights were considered "dominant" to losers.

In the first trial, thirty monkeys were divided into two groups. Half were placed in a chronically stressful, socially unstable milieu, and the other half were maintained in a nonstresful, socially stable invironment. Both groups were given a high-cholesterol, high-fat diet.

After 22 months, the dominant aggressive and competitive monkeys in the chronically stressed, socially disrupted groups developed artery blockages twice as severe as the dominant monkeys in the unstressed group. The dominant, stressed monkeys also had twice as much blockage as monkeys in the subordinate groups who did not fight. These differences in artery blockages occurred even though blood pressure and cholesterol levels were comparable in all groups.

In a second study, the experimenters fed the monkeys a diet lower in fat. The monkeys developed fewer blockages than in the first trial, but the dominant, chronically stressed monkeys had significantly more blockages than the other groups of monkeys.

The authors concluded from their investigations that psychosocial influences on coronary artery atherosclerosis were not dependent on the presence of large amounts of fat and cholesterol in the diet. Stress caused formation of coronary artery blockages even when monkeys were fed low fat and low cholesterol. When the diet was higher in fat and cholesterol, the influence of stress in causing arterial blockages was magnified thirty times. Therefore, emotional stress was deemed to be the most powerful influence in the development of coronary artery blockages.

Although the study by Kaplan and colleagues (1982) was considered to be a pioneer study showing the best scientific evidence to date on the role of stress in body malfunctioning, the mind–body perspective is almost as old as human history.

A Brief Historical Review

To understand the mind–body perspective in depth and breadth, it is necessary to become familiar with some of the history of medical thought. In prehistoric times, illness and disease were seen as existing outside the person. It was alleged that forces such as ghosts attacked the individual and could only be dispelled through purging or exorcism (Sheridan and Kline 1984). Remnants of these ideas are still widespread.

Medicine from 2,500 to 500 B.C., during the Babylonia-Assyrian civilization, was dominated by religion, and suggestion was the major tool of treatment. In effect, a psychosomatic or mind–body perspective was the dominant motif for 2,000 years prior to the year 1 (Sigerist 1951).

Around 400 B.C. during the Greek civilization, Socrates

alleged that it was not "proper" to cure the eyes without the head, nor the head without the body. The founder of Western medicine, Hippocrates, around the same time, reported that fear produced sweat and that shame brought on palpitations of the heart. He equated health to a harmonious balance of mind, body, and the environment. However, in the Middle Ages, these observations were replaced by a return to the belief that malevolent powers and sin were the causes of illness. Such evil was seen as both inside and outside the sufferer and as a province of the church (Sheridan and Kline 1984).

After 1,000 years of religious dominance, interest in natural causes and cures of disease returned. The telescope and the microscope brought more of the unseen world into the domain of the observable and known. Knowledge regarding the soma multiplied and the psyche was pushed out of the field of scientific study (Freedman et al. 1976).

Although the Renaissance brought renewed interest in the scientific study of medicine, through the nineteenth century the mind–body schism spread to its furthest division. The study of the body was the province of science and the study of the psyche, often referred to as "the soul," was the province of the church. Psychological influences were considered "unscientific." "It became common to treat the disease and not the patient" (Freedman et al. 1976, p. 794).

Sigmund Freud's Contribution

It was Sigmund Freud who brought psyche and soma back together and demonstrated the importance of the emotions in producing both mental disturbances and somatic disorders.

Freud pulled the doctor-patient relationship out of the religious framework of hope and faith by emphasizing transference and countertransference (Freedman et al. 1976).

More than any contributor before him, Freud demonstrated how psychological factors caused bodily ills. Further, by helping his patients talk about their feelings, he could help them rid themselves of paralyses and other "hysterical conversion" symptoms such as hysterical blindness and deafness (Freud 1896, 1897). The results of his research were so convincing that some of his followers tried to explain all illness as an expression of repressed ideas or fantasies (Singer 1977).

Perhaps in his formulations of psychosexual development do we see Freud's attempts to integrate psychological and somatic functions at its clearest and best. In describing the developing child, Freud posited that to know what was of major concern to the child, the observer had to know what part of the body the child was cathecting—oral, anal or phallic, that is, the mouth, the anus, or the genitals. Furthermore, a psychoanalytic perspective on neuroses and other emotional dysfunctions always takes into consideration the patient's fantasies on oral, anal, and phallic wishes. Finally, Freud alleged that many of our daily activities are sublimations of biological functions. For example, reading and other forms of learning are viewed as derivative of the desire to eat, for example, a hunger for knowledge (Freud 1905a).

Other Contributors

Using Freud's insights, a number of workers in the early decades of the twentieth century tried to expand the understanding of the interrelationship of psyche and soma. Two trends developed, one suggesting that specific emotions tend to lead to specific cell and tissue damage, and the second holding that anxiety creates preconditions for a number of diseases (Freedman et al. 1976).

One of Freud's contemporaries, Wilhelm Reich (1949), centered much of his treatment on the patient's overt bodily tensions. He alleged that by calling attention to the patient's posture, use of the hands, facial contortions, and so forth, the patient would be able to get in touch with his or her basic wishes, fantasies, defenses, and emotions. This perspective is utilized to this day by many contemporary psychotherapists (Strean 1990).

Franz Alexander (1965) contended that if a specific stimulus or stress occurred, it expressed itself in a specific response of a predetermined organ. He applied Cannon's (1929, 1939) fight or flight concept to demonstrate how stress is handled. Alexander pointed out that when an individual experiences stress, he may repress the stressful ideas and emotions and produce through the voluntary nervous system a reaction similar to the hysterical conversion response described by Freud (1897). After repressing the stressful thoughts and feelings, the individual may, through his autonomic nervous system, keep his or her sympathetic responses alert for heightened aggression or flight. The individual may also arrange to keep his or her parasympathetic responses alerted for heightened vegetative activities. Alexander demonstrated that prolonged alertness and tension can produce physiological disorders and eventual pathology of the organs of the viscera.

One of Alexander's major contributions was his emphasis on the unresolved dependency conflicts of the psychosomatic patient. Unable to put into words his or her dependency yearnings, the patient "speaks through the body." For example, thoughts and feelings that cannot be stomached may be expressed by an ulcer. Frustrated yearnings for love may be manifested in heart difficulties, and unacceptable wishes to cling can result in a headache (Alexander 1965).

In formulating hypotheses on cardiovascular disturbances, Alexander (1939) did his most extensive work on hypertension. According to Alexander, there is in hypertension a continuous struggle against hostile impulses. The patient tends to inhibit aggressive and assertive wishes because he or she is apprehensive about losing the love and/or the presence of a loved object.

Earlier we referred to the work of W. B. Cannon and mentioned that Alexander was much influenced by him. Other workers interested in the mind–body interactions have also been assisted by Cannon's formulations. Cannon (1929, 1939) was one of the first to note that the body actually makes observable changes when the individual is in pain or experiences fear or rage. In discussing his "fight or flight" response–the internal adaptive response of the body to a threat–Cannon showed that the body secretes catecholamines, or "stress hormones," that immediately arouse key organs, preparing a person under threat to fight or run. Best known of these hormones is epinephrine, better known as adrenaline, which is produced by adrenal glands located just on top of each kidney.

As Kenneth Pelletier (1993) has pointed out in "Between Mind and Body: Stress, Emotions and Health," the fight or flight response was essential to survival in a time when human beings faced physical threats, such as from wild animals, which caused acute stress and could be dealt with by either fighting or running away. By contrast, the stresses we have to cope with in modern life are more likely to be psychological and interpersonal and therefore we cannot easily cope with them by fighting or fleeing. However, as Hans Selye (1950, 1978), a pioneering stress researcher at McGill University in Montreal, Canada, has demonstrated, the body reacts to contemporary stresses as if it were still trying to cope with a real physical danger.

Hans Selye (1950, 1978) coordinated a vast number of observations under the name of *general adaptation syndrome*. This term suggests a complex chain of events, initiated by a variety of stressful situations (stressors) and mediated by hormonal mechanisms. According to Selye's formulations, the first hormonal response to stress is the *alarm reaction*. In the case of prolonged stress, *chronic hormonal defensive reactions* ensue (the stage of resistance). It is these chronic and excessive hormonal changes, mediated primarily by the anterior pituitary and adrenal cortex, which lead to various pathological changes in end-organs and are designated as diseases of adaptation, for example, arthritis (*periarteritis nodosa*).

In *Mind as Healer, Mind as Slayer*, Pelletier (1992) pointed out that there are two forms of stress–short-term or acute, and long-term or chronic–and they have different consequences for health. If one is under chronic stress (for example, constant pressure of deadlines, major interpersonal difficulties with a boss or spouse), the body reacts with the same physical changes that would be appropriate if one were under acute stress (a close call on the highway or the reaction to a loud noise). Catecholamines trigger a series of physiological changes which marshal the body to readiness. Heart rate, blood pressure, and the blood level of glucose all rise sharply.

This physical turmoil usually goes along with anxiety and unpleasant thoughts.

Under conditions of chronic, long-term stress, the normal responses which occur under short-term stress are abnormally protracted and can lead to chronic disease or contribute to the development of disease. With chronic stress, the immune system tends to be suppressed and then the blood cholesterol level rises. When protracted over time, the normal short term increases in blood pressure can result in hypertension and increases in the heart rate. This can raise the risk of an arrhythmia.

An early contributor to the mind–body perspective was the English psychiatrist and psychoanalyst Edward Glover (1949). In contrast to Alexander who contended that psychosomatic disorders have specific content and meaning (for example, a lonely heart, a nervous stomach), Glover averred that psychosomatic disorders

> although influenced by psychic reactions at some point or another in their progress, have in themselves no psychic content, and consequently do not represent stereotyped patterns of conflict. Should they develop psychic meaning, it may be assumed that a psychoneurotic process has been superimposed on a psychosomatic foundation. [pp. 170-171]

Alexander's point of view as discussed in "The Psychosomatic Approach in Medicine," a chapter in the book *Dynamic Psychiatry* (Alexander and Ross 1952), has been supported by renowned writers such as Otto Fenichel (1945) and Flanders Dunbar (1943, 1944, 1947). Both paid much attention to the personality dynamics which are commonly found in patients with somatic dysfunctions. However, as we suggested at the beginning of this section, the controversy about whether or not psychosomatic illnesses can have specific psychological interpretations continues to this day.

Steward Wolff and Harold Wolff (1947) studied a number of physiological reactions under experimentally induced emotional states. In their study of "Tom," a man with gastric fistula, they made careful observations of gastric activity, together with specific physiological measurements, under varying life situations in response to experimentally induced emotional conditions. They made similar studies on the eye, on the mucous membranes of the colon, bronchi, nose, on patients with essential hypertension, and diabetes. H. Wolfin (1950) has interpreted many of these reactions as serving the purpose of warding off noxious stimuli. An illustration of such an interpretation is the following:

> Conspicuous among defensive protective reactions are those involving the nose and airways. It has been observed that in reaction to assaults and threat, certain individuals occlude their air passages and limit the ventilatory exchange by vasodilatation, turgescence, hypersecretion, and contraction of smooth and skeletal muscle. The changes, especially in the upper respiratory airways, give rise to a variety of symptoms, notably pain and obstruction, the latter often leading to secondary infection, and the prolongation of morbid processes. Also the individual exhibits a behavior pattern and attitude of a nonparticipation in interpersonal relations. [p.1075]

Wolfin's interpretation is essentially an extension of Cannon's (1929, 1939) orientation concerning the mechanisms of "fight or flight" to a great many physiological reactions not considered or accounted for by Cannon (Alexander 1952).

Engel (1950) used the term *syncope*, or fainting, and suggested that the symptom may be due to a variety of causes. He also pointed out that the underlying pathological processes which lead to syncope may be classified according to three basic mechanisms:

> 1. Altered cerebral metabolism due to circulatory disturbances; 2. Altered cerebral metabolism due to metabolic factors; 3. Psychological mechanisms not involving any known disturbance in cerebral metabolism or circulation. [p. 5]

According to Engel (1950) the two most common types of fainting in young adults are *vasodepressor* and *hysterical*. The physiological mechanism underlying vasodepressor syncope is that of a sudden fall in blood pressure. Although the fainting reaction my be initiated in any position, hypotension and unconsciousness are more likely to occur in the erect rather than in the recumbent position because of the effect of gravity. Psychologically, fainting of this type tends to occur in situations which induce fear and anxiety from real and imagined impending dangers. Usually the affects accompanying the fear and anxiety are repressed.

Engel (1962), based on his research, advanced the theory that psychosomatic phenomena might be avoided in cases where neurotic organizations have arisen. The latter, he suggested, will form a "buffering function" between mind and body. In effect, the psyche creates a protective structure in the form of a neurotic symptom to deal with psychological conflict and therefore prevents somatic eruptions.

Similar to Engel's (1962) perspective was Lidz's (1959). In a chapter in *American Handbook of Psychiatry* (Arieti 1959) entitled "General Concepts of Psychosomatic Medicine," Lidz was able to demonstrate that the person who is prey to psychosomatic illness has suffered serious insecurity early in life

> but has not erected adequate mechanisms of defense to protect against the danger. Rather, he avoids recurrence of the insecurity or trauma by patterning his life so that he will never be exposed again. The critical area of weakness is encapsulated, but the patient neither becomes desensitized to the insecurity nor develops mechanisms of defense to blunt its impact. [p. 652]

Jurgen Rensch (1948), who has utilized communication theory to explain psychosomatic problems, concluded that the person with a psychosomatic disease has not developed the adult processes of communication through words and gestures. Instead, he has remained at a level of communication which an immature child utilizes–the use of the body.

Melitta Sperling (1949, 1950, 1952) was one of the first clinicians to discuss in depth the psychodynamics and treatment of the psychosomatic patient. Like others who preceded her (for example, Alexander 1939, 1952, Reich 1949), Sperling suggested that the individual suffering from psychosomatic problems defends strongly against recognizing dependency yearnings. By utilizing the mechanisms of denial and reaction formation, these mechanisms have become ingrained in the individual's character structure since childhood.

For psychotherapy with the psychosomatic patient, Sperling (1952) suggested that "similar to the reaction of the latent psychotic patient, in whom the removal of neurotic defenses can produce an acute psychotic episode, so in the psychosomatic the analysis of the very strong reaction formation can bring about the aggravation of the patient's somatic condition" (p. 289).

Sperling (1949, 1950, 1952) repeatedly warned that the clinician working with the psychosomatic patient in psychotherapy must understand that "cure" has not been effected when the symptom has been removed.

> Not only is treatment of the disease not finished then; it has actually not even begun. The repressed impulses which had formerly found expression in the symptom may now break through in a behavior problem.... [The clinician] must understand that by clearing up a somatic symptom he has not touched the cause of the disease, and that the disease will break out in another symptom, or in a recurrence of the old symptom, or in a behavior problem, or in some other manifestation, whenever the patient's infantile dependency needs are frustrated, unless these dependency needs are resolved psychoanalytically. [1952, p. 292]

A contemporary of Sperling, and one of Freud's personal physicians, Max Schur (1951) concluded that most structural changes in organs of the body have a psychological component. He also contended that the psychosomatic patient has conflicts which originated in the preverbal period of development, that is, when dependency yearnings were at their greatest (and were responded to ambivalently). Schur pointed out that the psychosomatic patient cannot translate his reactions "into *our* language; it would have to be translated into the language of an infant" (p. 247).

By the late 1960s and early 1970s the mind–body perspective was becoming more ·popular and increasingly more accepted by physicians, psychotherapapists, and the general community (Engel 1967, Lerner and Noy 1968, Reiser 1966, Von Bertalanffy 1964, Winnicott 1966, Wittkower 1969). In an article, "Psychosomatic Disorders," Sternschein (1975) in describing the state of the art, quoted Lord Chesterfield, the English statesman and writer, who said, "I find, by experience, that the mind and body are more than married, for they are most intimately united; and when one suffers, the other sympathizes" (p. 374). Sternschein, though acknowledging that the psyche and soma always play interdependent roles in all illnesses, cautioned that patients need considerable help in being sensitized to this important notion.

In 1978, Nemiah introduced the concept of *alexithymia*. This refers to the discovery that we have alluded to several times in this chapter, namely, that certain individuals do not have words to describe their emotional states, either because they are unaware of them or because they are incapable of distinguishing one emotion from another. For example, they may not be able to distinguish anxiety from depression, excitement from fatigue, or anger from hunger (McDougall 1989).

During the last two decades there has been a developing literature consistently demonstrating that beliefs, thoughts, and emotions do create chemical reactions which uphold life in every cell. Further, there is now limited doubt that if thoughts and feelings create anxiety and stress, the bodily functions will be negatively affected and can deteriorate (Benson 1976, Charash 1991, Chopra 1993, Cortis 1995, Cousins 1983, 1989, Lazare 1987, Lynch 1985, McDougall 1989, Nicholson 1995, Ornish 1990, Patlack 1994, Pelletier 1992, Sacks 1995). Not only do we now have scientific evidence showing that depression can actually compromise the effectiveness of disease-fighting cells in the immune system (Goleman and Gurin 1993) but we also know that a human relationship which inspires hope and offers love and laughter can combat serious diseases (Cousins 1989).

Although the general effects of stress on the body have been known for decades, currently we are very much aware that psychological factors play a crucial role in determining whether people subjected to stressful events will get sick or not. A growing number of studies indicate that mind-body approaches can help prevent or treat many diseases related to lifestyle (Pelletier 1993).

Concomitant with the mind–body perspective becoming increasingly acceptable to professionals and non-professionals alike, the relationship of the brain and heart has been under serious examination. Let us now turn to some of the major notions and hypotheses that are inherent in the brain–heart perspective.

The Brain–Heart Perspective

A sentiment which has been attributed to Aristotle avers that the heart is the seat of life and the origin of all emotions. Whether Aristotle's statement is valid or not, no one questions the fact that the heart is the organ of the body to which we refer daily in order to describe our emotions and our emotional states. When we are in a heated discussion or debate, we want to get to "the heart of the matter," implying that the heart is the essence of what we are talking about. A presidential candidate concluded that he won the election because he used the slogan, "In your heart you know he's right," suggesting that by listening to the voices resonating from the heart one will get to the real truth. A basketball coach, mournfully discussing his team's loss, said, "They played their hearts out," suggesting that the team members gave everything to try to win the game. A student who did extremely well on an examination, asked how she prepared for the exam, replied, "I knew everything by heart," meaning that she had mastered and memorized every fact and figure in the text.

Our everyday language is replete with metaphors which involve the heart. Furthermore, most of us find that when the heart is utilized in conversation, the meaning is usually quite clear. The following are expressions which do not need much, if any, explanation or translation: "My heart isn't in it." "I was heartbroken." "I wish you wouldn't be so hard-hearted." "I heartily endorse your plan." "You have my heartfelt sympathy."

Very often the heart emerges as a person. We speak of a "raging heart," a "hungry heart," and a "sweetheart." A heart can be "full" or "empty." We can "pour our hearts out" or "eat our hearts out." And, we can become "heartsick" or not have "enough heart."

There has been an intuitive notion persisting for many centuries that the heart is the seat of life; yet, it is only recently that scientific evidence has been available to affirm the notion.

As we said earlier in this chapter, it has been repeatedly demonstrated that emotional stress may be accompanied by measurable changes in arterial blood pressure, heart rate, stroke volume, and cardiac output (Alexander 1939, Ax 1953, Reiser and Bakst 1959, Schacter 1957). One of the most thorough studies is that of Hickam and colleagues (1948), who utilized a spontaneous nonspecific stress situation—an important college examination—in order to demonstrate differences in measurements reflecting circulatory dynamics obtained during "tension" from measurements obtained during relative relaxation.

Twenty-three "healthy" medical students served as subjects in the study. Each student was examined just before the examination and then a day later, after being informed of passing the examination. The average cardiac index (volume output of the heart in liters per minute per square meter body surface area) before the examination was two liters per minute per square meter greater than that measured during relative relaxation. When the figure was converted to "work load," it corresponded to a load which would be demanded by increasing oxygen consumption by an amount equal to the basal metabolism.

In the work of Hickam and colleagues (1948) (as well as that of the authors mentioned above), the meaning of the stress and the nature of the stress reaction were not specifically studied on an individualized basis. However, Hickam did note that the pattern of mobilization varied in his subjects, and he described three patterns. For most of the group, anxiety was accompanied by an increase in cardiac index, decrease in peripheral resistance, and a small rise in mean arterial pressure. In a smaller second group, the "anxious state" was associated with a slight to moderate rise in blood pressure and peripheral resistance, and no change in the cardiac index.

Studies by Ax (1953), Funkenstein and colleagues (1953), and Schacter (1957) who worked with subjects in laboratory situations deliberately staged to evoke either anxiety or hostility, reported differences in patterns of circulatory changes. Specifically these studies affirmed that outwardly displayed anger is accompanied by a release of norepinephrine, whereas anxiety and anger directed inward are accompanied by a release of epinephrine.

It has continually been found that stressful life events often precede the development of episodes of congestive heart failure (Cortis 1995, Reiser and Bakst 1959). Reiser and Bakst (1959) interviewed twenty-five consecutive patients who were admitted to the wards of the Cincinnati General Hospital because of congestive heart failure. An acute emotionally stressful experience had immediately preceded the development of congestive failure in 76 percent of the cases. In each instance, these events seemed to have highly specific meaning for the patient in relation to his previous life experiences and conflicts, and in most cases they were superimposed upon a chronic state of emotional tension. Marked improvement in clinical status coincided with providing the patient with an opportunity to share and discuss his difficulties with a physician. It was further observed that a continuing supportive relationship with the physician aided in avoiding further unresolved emotional crises and stabilized the clinical course to a great extent. This type of intervention and its success has been demonstrated by many researchers many times up to the present (Benson 1976, Chopra 1993, Cortis 1995, Cousins 1976, 1983, Grinker and Robbins 1954, Lynch 1985, Ornish 1990).

Reiser and Bakst (1959) were among the first to identify

several psychological burdens imposed by the onset and/or diagnosis of heart disease. These burdens may stem from any or all of three general sources:

> The first source is constituted by the symptoms themselves. The abrupt onset of sensations such as breathlessness, severe precordial pain, palpitation, dizziness, etc. is in itself understandably terrifying...
>
> The second source is the threat inherent in the diagnosis of heart disease. Any illness may generate anxiety by virtue of actual or threatened damage to bodily integrity, but in the case of the heart these issues are exquisitely exaggerated. The reasons for this are general and universal. The central indispensable role of the heart in maintaining life provides an appropriate background for the use of its mental representation as a symbolic object of the deepest and most awesome unconscious fantasy fears of all types....It is probable that the diagnosis of heart disease universally activates, to some degree, fantasies of sudden, unexpected, and catastrophic death....The unconscious threat may be no less intense in the patient who is informed of the discovery of a functional cardiac murmur than it is in a patient confronted by a diagnosis of serious advanced rheumatic heart disease....
>
> The third source of anxiety stems from the fact that the patient experiences a real limitation of his physical capacity and [worries] that this will be progressive and result in increasing loss of power in his most vital organ. [Reiser and Bakst 1959, pp. 665-666]

As many writers report (Cortis 1995, Cousins 1983, Reiser and Bakst 1959), defenses such as denial (of the heart disease) or reaction formation (against dependent wishes) may lead to unrealistic and rebellious unwillingness to adhere to a prescribed medical regime.

Many other defenses which were adaptive in the past may become maladaptive when the patient confronts the reality of heart disease and needs to rely on these defenses more because of his or her increased anxiety. For example, the habitual use of projection can intensify and the patient then becomes increasingly paranoid. He or she may begin to view the spouse or colleagues as enemies. As the heart disease becomes more of a reality, the patient may wish to regress and can become very demanding on those around. Then individuals in his or her social orbit are alienated and a vicious cycle takes place whereby the heart patient feels unloved and isolated and this has a realistic basis (Cousins 1983, Reiser and Bakst 1959).

As the patient sees himself or herself more as an invalid, the self image and body image also alter and secondary gains increase. The patient begins to feel that because his major organ, the heart, is inferior, he or she is inferior (Adler 1967).

Emotional Aspects of Cardiac Surgery

As we suggested earlier in this chapter, bypass surgery has many limitations. What has not been sufficiently considered is that the acute anxiety engendered by just the suggestion of heart surgery can lead to increased damage to the heart. As we know, when anxiety is not relieved, the heart does not work well. But, insufficient concern has been given to how to discuss the idea of heart surgery and what impact verbal interventions have on the vulnerable patient. In addition, the surgery itself often activates serious psychological problems.

Fox and colleagues (1954), having been impressed by the large number of requests for psychiatric consultations by the cardiac surgical service in a general hospital, undertook a study of psychological reactions of patients right before their surgeries. These researchers reported a high incidence of serious psychological problems (for example, acute anxiety reactions, incessant crying, intense obsessive preoccupation) before and after the surgery. In 1955, Bliss and colleagues, having encountered two patients who developed severe schizophrenic psychoses after mitral commissurotomy, did a retrospective study of thirty-seven cases and reported that eleven of them had developed "major psychiatric complications." Kaplan (1956) studied eighteen patients who also had experienced mitral commissurotomy and stressed the importance of the individual personality structure and life situation as determinants of the ways in which these people responded to improved cardiac function.

In 1957, Priest and his colleagues, confronted with a higher incidence of psychoses after cardiac surgery than after general major surgery, studied a large group of patients undergoing heart operations. They emphasized the uniformly high degree of anxiety in cardiac patients approaching surgery and related this to the disproportionately high incidence of psychiatric complications. They drew attention to the difficulty in evaluating surgical results because of the postoperative persistence of psychological symptoms such as fatigue, insomnia, and chronic tension.

Helene Deutsch (1965) pointed out that the heart patient's history, particularly how he or she experienced previous operations and illnesses, will always tend to influence perceptions in the present. Stated Deutsch,

> I have noted, for example, that operations performed in childhood leave indelible traces on the psychic life of the individual. Memories or affective reactions to the original operation return again and again in certain situations. The reaction to an operation later in life corresponds often in form and essence to that of the first. [pp. 287-288]

In her research, Deutsch also noted that common to most, if not all, heart patients was the fact that the operation mobilized a large amount of aggression, whose motives and fate have an individual character. In addition, common to all patients facing some form of heart surgery is that the patient, if a woman, has fantasies that the surgery is a delivery, and if a man "castration stands in the center of the experience" (Deutsch 1965, p. 289). Many psychotherapists have reported (for example, Lindermann 1941, Menninger 1934) that in their dreams and associations to operations, men were fighting with another man or with a group of men.

Deutsch (1965) was one of the first researchers to remind physicians, particularly those who do surgery, to be aware of and sensitive to the psychic life of the heart patient. She also felt that the physicians' "own psychic make-up" plays an important role in the heart patient's recovery or lack of it.

The Psychological Component of Heart Disease Grows in Importance

For the past three decades, those professionals involved in the treatment and prevention of heart disease have become increasingly sensitized to the emotional factors which contribute toward heart disease and to those psychological factors which must be addressed in order to reverse it.

In the mid-'50s, Grinker and Robbins (1954) demonstrated that the increased tempo of life in contemporary Western civilization multiplied the stresses which directly affected cardiac musculature and the coronary vessels. They noted that precordial pain was a frequent symptom of middle-aged, active individuals in our culture.

By the mid-'50s, heart disease was so frequent that many individuals who suffered from precordial pain observed members of their families suffering from cardiac disease or dying from coronary insufficiency. It was discovered then that certain psychological conflicts in relation to those who have died from coronary disease can induce identical pains in otherwise healthy individuals, as though the healthy individuals were subjected to the same stressful conditions as their relatives. Thus, neurotic cardiac pains are frequently a symptom in individuals whose parents have a history of coronary disease (Arlow 1952, Grinker and Robbins 1954).

In the '50s, the psychodynamics of the person suffering from heart disease began to be more discussed and assessed. The most frequent conflict noted was between oral, dependency wishes and a hostile, aggressive attitude toward the same person (Alexander 1952, Grinker and Robbins 1954). When oral demands from and rage toward the same significant person appear together, even though unconsciously, the physiological effects may be the simultaneous stimulation of the vagus and the sympathetic nerves. The increased demands from sympathetic stimulation at the time that there is a chronic vagal effect on the heart may produce coronary spasm and deficient oxygenation of the muscles, resulting in much pain (Grinker and Robbins 1954).

The first definitive text on the psychodynamics and psychotherapeutic treatment of heart disease was written by Daniel Schneider in 1967. Stressing the strong relationship between the brain and the heart, Schneider emphasized that the "coronary personality who is always in a hurry" is constantly coping with intense rage that he is busy trying to repress. Leading a very stressful life, the coronary personality is always dealing with "the weight of stress, the deep root of childhood terror and horror and unspeakable humiliation–a veritable pyramid of burdens to the heart [which] are elements to conjure with in every case. Any and every human being is subject to their impact as shock" (p. xi).

Many subsequent researchers who have been interested in the psychological components of heart disease have replicated Schneider's findings on the role of rage in heart problems. States Schneider:

> We can become enraged when we are being forced to accept or to be humiliated by a hated and hostile object. If we cannot retaliate, we must "swallow rage".... All of this has to do not merely with being conquered but also with being subjugated...much as beasts are harnessed. The feeling of rage can be summarized as one in which we are in the most violent recoil against being forced without justice and in the most hurtful and humiliating manner to a status, somewhat less than human, forced down a regressive path....
>
> Rage, the emotion provoked as an aftermath of psychic injury, always threatens the heart. [pp. 104-105]

A study showing the link between personality dynamics and heart disease was the work by Friedman and Rosenman on the Type A syndrome. Although the authors began their research in the 1950s, Friedman and Rosenman published *Type A Behavior and Your Heart* in 1981, and *Treating Type A Behavior and Your Heart* in 1984. The Type A syndrome describes an individual who is hostile, self-involved, impatient, cynical, and always in a hurry. These individuals make compulsive attempts to achieve lofty goals and have a strong wish to receive recognition and advancement. They have a tendency to want to do many things at once, such as talking and moving quickly.

Scherwitz and colleagues (1978) and Williams (1989), in separate studies, demonstrated that the factors most toxic to the heart are self-involvement, hostility, and cynicism.

A study endorsed by most experts treating heart disease is that by Lynch (1985). In *The Language of the Heart*, Lynch was able to demonstrate that those who suffered from heart disease usually felt "socially isolated." Experts such as Ornish (1990) and Cortis (1995) concurred with Lynch that anything that promotes a sense of isolation leads to chronic stress and therefore to heart disease. Conversely, as Ornish (1990) states: "Anything that leads to real intimacy and feelings of connection can be healing in the real sense of the word.... The ability to be intimate has long been seen as a key to emotional health; I believe it is essential to the health of our hearts as well" (p. 87).

Numerous studies in the last decade (for example, Ornish 1990, Scherwitz 1978, Williams 1989) all conclude that the self-involvement, hostility, and cynicism that predispose people to heart disease are really effects of a more fundamental cause—the perception of isolation.

Although the research to date on the relationship of personality dynamics to heart disease has been flourishing, limited in-depth studies have been conducted. For example, why is the Type A personality impatient and self-involved? Why do individuals with oral dependency problems get angry so frequently? What is it about social support that reverses heart disease? Is the laughter that accompanies it a factor? Although most experts agree that stress is an inevitable variable in heart disease, what is stress? These and other questions will be subjected to intensive examination in the pages ahead.

LIBRARY, UNIVERSITY COLLEGE CHESTER

2

Stressing
the Heart

One of the many informal research projects on heart disease which I conducted over a period of one year was interviewing heart patients and their family members. This occurred in many different settings—hospitals, homes, offices, and restaurants. I asked them about their subjective views on the causes and treatment of heart disease. One question that I repeatedly posed to my subjects was, "What do you regard as the most significant thing that caused your (or your spouse's, parent's, and so forth) heart problems? The following is a random sampling of the many responses I received:

A 70-year-old psychologist, who had a mild heart attack a month before I asked the question, replied, "My daughter's serious illness upset me very much and her illness still has not left my mind."

A 40-year-old stockbroker told me that three weeks after he was informed that his mother had a short time to live, he had a massive heart attack.

"When I hit my sixtieth birthday, I went into a depression and shortly afterward I developed chest pains and shortness of breath. The angiogram showed I had arteries that were very clogged," commented an advertising executive.

A 49-year-old housewife who developed a severe heart condition informed me that she noted that when her "last child" went off to college and she was "all alone" with her husband, she felt her "heart was broken."

An attorney of 67 years who just had his second heart attack within a five year period commented, "I'm not as powerful these days and I've always been very competitive. I think that ever since I learned that I couldn't win them all, I've been heartsick."

The husband of a 40-year-old woman who "needed" a quadruple bypass told me, "You see, we were talking seriously about divorce and I think it really affected her."

A 55-year-old psychotherapist told me, "I used to be very successful. My practice was going downhill. I felt increasingly angry and agitated and then came the heart attack."

One of the most obvious themes in the responses is that all of the respondents attributed heart problems to interpersonal events that induced sadness, anger, and agitation. Although my sample of over 100 did not adhere to strict statistical standards, I strongly believe that it is not chance that almost all respondents believed heart problems were caused by psychological conflicts that could not be mastered. My random sampling also tends to validate the many empirical studies we discussed in Chapter 1 which offered scientific evidence of the role of emotional conflict in heart disease (for example, Cortis 1995, Ornish 1990, Reiser and Bakst 1959).

In discussing heart problems with colleagues, fellow-patients, patients of mine in psychotherapy, and friends, I found that the most frequently used term in referring to the etiology of heart problems was *stress*. Repeatedly I have heard statements like: "Stress was my downfall." "His heart attack came after he was under a lot of stress." "Avoid stress and you'll avoid a heart attack."

Although any content analysis of a heart disease discussion demonstrates that "stress" is the modal term regardless of the setting of the discussion, the age and sex of the respondents, and the nature of the heart problems, it is not clear what professionals and nonprofessionals really mean by "stress." Whenever I have asked someone to define the term, I have never received a clear answer. In addition, I have struggled many times over long periods without coming up with a satisfactory answer to "What is stress?"

Defining Stress

Despite the fact that many, if not most, writers on heart disease utilize the term "stress" and offer all kinds of evidence to demonstrate that stress "causes" or is "definitely linked" to heart disease, very few of them define the term. Kenneth Pelletier (1993), in his article "Between Mind and Body: Stress, Emotions and Health," stated: "Although we all know what stress is when we experience it, coming to grips with it scientifically has been a major challenge. One problem is that the very definition of stress has been vague and inconsistent, sometimes referring to an outside force, sometimes to the body's reaction to it" (p. 26). Pelletier mentions in his article that early in 1986, several private foundations funded a major conference in Tucson, Arizona, of psychologists, immunologists, and physicians. They met to define a common ground in terminology, research procedures, and measurement in the area of psychoneuroimmunology. Ironically, the first stumbling block was an attempt to define stress, which "led to the unanimous conclusion that any absolute definition was literally impossible" (p. 27).

When researchers refer to being "under stress," they usually imply what the dictionary definition of the term suggests: being "under stress" implies being "under pressure" (Winston Dictionary 1943). However, where there is a lack of concurrence and clarity among the writers is where the pressure is coming from.

In trying to determine where "the pressure" or "stress" is coming from, I believe it is important to differentiate between "stressors," which are stimuli which impinge on an individual, and "stress," which is an idiosyncratic, subjective experience. Examples of stressors may be divorce, death in the family, loss of a job, pregnancy, or being caught in a traffic jam.

Rahe (1975) in "Epidemiological Studies of Life Change and Illness," developed a classic, systematized method of quantifying stressors and correlating the event in people's lives with their illnesses. He showed that the more stress a person experienced, the more likely it was that he or she would become sick over the next several months. Rahe established the notion of "life change units" (LCUs) and gave them numerical equivalents. For example, a divorce is equivalent to 38 LCUs, while being fired from work is equivalent to 64 LCUs.

Although most researchers on stress tend to emphasize "stressors" and appear compatible with Rahe's perspective, this approach has a serious limitation. It bypasses the individual's subjective interpretations of the external event, the unique conflicts it arouses, and the strength or weakness of his or her defense mechanisms and other coping devices. For example, when Arthur, a man in his early forties, was told by his wife of four years that she was going to divorce him, he felt humiliated, devastated, and became very depressed. Two months later he had a massive heart attack. By contrast, Bertha, a woman in her middle thirties, on finalizing a divorce from her husband of five years, felt very relieved and referred to her mood as "being ecstatic." To allocate the same LCUs to Arthur and Bertha would be a serious mistake. Each of these individuals has to be separately assessed to note the quality and quantity of stress that each experiences.

What we have cautioned about a stressor such as divorce would be applicable to other stressors such as job loss, physical injury, financial difficulties, and so forth. For example, some individuals feel deeply crushed on losing a job while others can feel enhanced, or at least relieved.

Florence Hollis (1972), a social work educator and researcher, distinguished between "press" and "stress." She viewed "the press" as an external variable that disrupts the individual's psychic equilibrium. How the person reacts to the press is what she referred to as "the stress."

Hans Selye (1978), whom we cited in Chapter 1, produced a large number of studies which have given support to the contention that stress is a biological reactive potentiality in all living organisms—a dynamic interplay of hormonal-metabolic responses within the organism to a wide variety of stimuli. In doing so he was careful to differentiate a "stimulus" which is an agent that predominantly stimulates a person to unique activity (Selye and Heuser 1955). Although his conceptual framework is essentially a biological one, his notion of keeping stimuli (or stressors) separate from the individual's unique activity is helpful in trying to define and clarify what stress is.

Accompaniments of Stress

In Chapter 1 we concluded that under the impact of strong emotions the body releases adrenalin into the blood stream. Adrenalin increases breathing and heartbeat rates as well as blood pressure. Cholesterol counts are raised and the demands on the heart and blood vessels are also exacerbated (Kunz and Finkel 1987). Other bodily symptoms have been designated as "symptoms of stress" by Pelletier (1993). These are stiff or tense muscles, grinding teeth, sweating, tension headaches, faint feelings, choking, difficulty in swallowing, stomachache, nausea, vomiting, loose bowels, constipation, frequency and urgency of urination, loss of interest in sex, tiredness, shakiness or tremors, and weight loss or gain.

Psychological symptoms of stress which have been noted (Flannery 1990, Pelletier 1993) are: anxious thoughts, fearful anticipation, poor concentration, difficulty with memory, irritability, restlessness, and difficulties in interpersonal relationships.

Although listing symptoms of stress gets us a step closer to the subjective experience of stress, it does not clarify just what the experience is or what causes it.

Stress—An Inability to Cope

As I have listened carefully to patients who have discussed in detail their unique reactions to "stressors" or "presses," I have tried to extract some common themes from their sessions so that the stress experience could be better understood. (I have also reflected many times on my own subjective reactions when I have experienced stress.)

Turning to the short vignettes at the beginning of the chapter, what all of the individuals experienced was an inability to master tasks and cope with life in their habitual ways. When I tuned in to the subjective states of mind of these individuals, and to other patients and colleagues of mine who were having difficulty coping with stressors, in almost every instance self-confidence and self-esteem were lowered, danger, though vague, was always in the air, and a feeling that one was being dominated by forces or individuals they could not control was almost always present.

Whenever I have put myself in the shoes of those unable to cope with a stressor like divorce, illness, or job loss, I inevitably feel the anger that the person in stress is experiencing. Often the anger is not overtly expressed, but a person in stress is rarely smiling, usually appears helpless and hopeless, and frequently feels unsupported.

Lazarus and Folkman (1984) defined the experience of stress as a state of discomfort when our problems exceed our resources to cope with them. What these writers imply is that the experience of stress is one in which we do not feel we are masters of our own fate. Our problems control us and we do not emotionally accept this ugly fact.

In sum, when we experience stress we experience a feeling of unknown danger, we do not feel we have the internal and/or external resources to cope with the problems that beset us. We are angry and feel dominated, helpless and hopeless. Usually we have lost our self-confidence, our self-esteem is lowered, and our sense of humor is gone.

A common occurrence which frequently stresses most of us is being caught in a traffic jam when we have to make an important appointment on time. As we sensitize ourselves to our emotional reactions to this universal stressor, we are usually angry because we cannot control our situation—the traffic controls us. We feel a danger is in the air but cannot be sure what punishments will accrue as we fantasize ourselves arriving late to the appointment. Inasmuch as we cannot master the task of moving in the traffic, we begin to doubt ourselves and find it difficult to like ourselves. We lose our sense of humor and continue to feel more helpless and hopeless.

One of the universal characteristics of the stress experience is that we do not accept the reality of the situation we are in. We do not say, "Okay, I'm in a traffic jam and that's the way it is." We are furious because we feel it should not be.

The inability to accept the reality of the stressor as a fact of life has important implications for understanding and treating heart disease. As we will discuss in more detail in the next section of this chapter, individuals with heart disease experience a great deal of stress because they often find themselves upset about situations they cannot change, such as income, family life, social status, achievement, and so forth (Flannery 1990, Ornish 1990).

Causes of Stress

In attempting to understand the major causes of stress, we will examine two crucial variables: the culture and the personality. It is well known that certain societal contexts induce more stress than others. We also know that certain personality types are more prone to experience a great deal of stress while others are stress-resistant. Let us first consider some of the cultural factors involved in the stress experience.

Our Stressful Culture

A 1987 Harris poll found that 89 percent of all Americans cited stress as a major problem in their lives. By stress these individuals meant that they felt unable to manage their daily lives comfortably and were proceeding at such a fast pace that most of the time they felt overwhelmed (Flannery 1990).

Ornish (1990) has related the chronic emotional stress of the 1990s to "the pace of life in the past ten years [which] seems to be increasingly faster—the so-called acceleration syndrome" (p.73). He further noted that like Alice in Wonderland, we go faster and faster while remaining in the same place. Federal Express overnight service is no longer quick enough. Even the traditional places of refuge in the twentieth century—the car and the home—are transformed, with fax machines and computers at home, telephones in the car, even fax machines for the car. Ornish concluded that our culture is one in which we often do not have time to recover from one stressful situation before we get hit with another. He reminds us that when our stress mechanisms are chronically activated, the same responses that are designed to protect us can become harmful—even lethal. Arteries constrict not just in our arms and legs but also inside our hearts, and blood clots are more likely to form inside our coronary arteries.

In discussing our cultural climate, it may be helpful to

differentiate between acute stress and chronic stress. Acute stress, it will be recalled, is prompted by an unexpected event that is perceived as a challenge to our sense of well-being and we feel that we are essentially not in control of the situation. This experience creates an alarm reaction characterized by sweating and rapid heartbeat (Cortis 1995). Examples of acute stress might involve being in a car accident or falling down on an icy street. Adrenaline causes blood to be directed toward the muscles, preparing us to fight or flee.

In contrast to short-term or acute stress, chronic stress is less adaptive and can be harmful. Long-term stress occurs when we experience a loss of control over ourselves and the environment. We experience a sense of failure and entrapment. The trapped energy is destructive to our hearts and can lead to chronically elevated blood pressure, augmented deposits of cholesterol in the arteries, and depression of the immune system. Examples of chronic stress are a conflicted marriage, lack of social support, an unhappy job situation, or continually finding no time to rest (Cortis 1995).

In our highly competitive culture where we are chronically ambitious and driven, chronic stress is inevitable. Few of us easily accept life as it is. Most of us want much more than we have and are constantly struggling to do much better.

When our goals are many and aspirations high, we are bound to feel constantly disappointed and deprived. Consequently, we are apt to feel very angry much of the time. Reuben Fine (1990) has referred to our society as "a hate culture" and has pointed out that most individuals harbor a great deal of distrust and suspicion in their interpersonal relationships. Competition is more valued than cooperation, and there is more self-centeredness than genuine concern for others.

In an attempt to unify psychology and the study of culture, Kardiner (1945) contributed the term *basic personality structure* to designate a group of character traits in the modal individual of a particular culture. Similar to Reuben Fine's (1990) findings, Kardiner concluded that the character traits most predominant in American culture are ambitiousness and greed.

A manifestation of "the hate culture" in which we reside is the divorce epidemic in this country where we have one divorce for every two marriages. Of marriages that sustain themselves, many can be characterized as full of one-upmanship fracases and pervasive friction (Strean 1995a). The "battered woman" syndrome is now a well known clinical entity and in *Wife Beating: The Silent Crisis*, Langley and Levy (1977) reported that one fifth of the married women in America beat their husbands but that few of the men would admit it. All of this helps us understand better why many married individuals experience chronic stress!

The idea that the family is a stable and cohesive unit in which father serves as economic provider and mother serves as emotional caregiver is a myth, according to Judith Bruce (1995), author of a study issued by the Population Council, an international nonprofit group based in New York that studies reproductive health. The study, "Families in Focus," found that all of the following are on an upswing: unwed motherhood, rising divorce rates, single parents taking care of children, and physical abuse.

Christopher Lasch (1978) has referred to our society as "the culture of narcissism"—a culture where we emphasize "Me first," and "I, I, I" seems to be our favorite subject matter. Here it is pertinent to point out that in the findings by Scherwitz and colleagues (1978), the frequency with which a person referred to himself or herself, that is, how frequently he or she used the words "I," "me," "my," and "mine" in an ordinary conversation actually predicted the recurrence of a heart attack. The more frequently an individual used those words, the greater likelihood he or she would die from a heart attack. Scherwitz also learned that people who use frequent self references later developed heart disease more often than people who did not. Furthermore, she discovered that there was an even greater degree of self-involvement in those who died from heart attacks.

Herbert Hendin (1975) has dubbed our current era "The Age of Sensation," in which people want what they want when they want it and get furious when they do not get it. He suggests that disruptive family life seems to reflect a cultural trend toward replacing commitment, involvement, and tenderness with self-aggrandizement, exploitativeness, and titillation. As other authors (for example, Coles 1975, Glick 1977, Strean 1994b) have also suggested, we now live in an age where we have unlimited expectations, many of us fantasize that Paradise can be regained and that the Garden of Eden can be relocated. There seems to be a rejection of feeling, commitment, and involvement. Individualism expresses itself in much egocentricity and impulse-ridden behavior. Glick (1977) has effectively demonstrated how increased narcissism has been tearing the family apart, and the tremendous value placed on "doing one's thing" has fostered the demise of the family unit. Because we want so very much that which is unrealistic, our frustration turns to desperation and our anguish becomes converted into heart disease (Cortis 1995).

Validating such notions on narcissism, sensationalism, individualism, and impulsiveness, Redford Williams (1989) showed how our society fosters heart disease. In his book *The Trusting Heart,* Williams demonstrated that the factors most toxic to the heart are self-involvement, hostility, and cynicism.

Over the decades psychological terms have been utilized to describe our current societal preoccupations. We have moved from the age of anxiety to the age of narcissism. Then came the age of sensationalism, and then the age of uncertainty. Perhaps we are headed toward the age of heartlessness?

Personality Type and Stress

As we discussed in Chapter 1, there are certain personality types who seek out pressuring situations, experience considerable stress, and therefore are more vulnerable to heart disease. Friedman and Rosenman's (1981, 1984) Type A personality is certainly one of these personality types. This individual, it will be recalled, is hostile, self-involved, impatient, and always in a hurry. He or she makes compulsive attempts to achieve poorly defined goals and has a strong desire for advancement and recognition. Driven, frustrated, pressured by deadlines and unable to relax, the Type A person nurtures past hurts and in many ways considers the world an unsafe place. As the Type A endlessly tries to control others, he or she reacts to minor hurts with harsh criticism of both the self and others. Constantly experiencing stress, the Type A person usually has high blood pressure and a high cholesterol count (Chopra 1993).

In *Heart and Soul,* Cortis (1995) quotes an article about physicians with heart disease: "The outstanding feature was the incessant treadmill of practice. Every one of these men had an additional factor, worry; in not a single case under fifty years of age was this feature absent" (p. 83). This unreferenced quote was published in 1924, describing a group of physicians who were sick in 1910. Thirty years later Flanders Dunbar (1944) described patients with coronary artery disease and used terms such as "compulsive," "a tendency to work long hours," "not take vacations," and had a "dislike of sharing responsibility." Cortis suggests that both quotations could apply to most people with heart disease today. They are Type A personalities who

> ...still seem to get more than their share of heart disease. Although everyone is different, the Type A person is involved in a chronic struggle to achieve more and more in less and less time. Type A behavior can cause physical damage in several ways. It can increase cholesterol level, blood pressure, and the likelihood of developing diabetes. Not surprisingly, Type A people are often cigarette smokers, which only makes their health problems worse. [Cortis 1995, p. 83]

Most writers who have discussed Type A behavior (for example, Charash 1991, Cortis 1995, Flannery 1990, Ornish 1990) emphasize the individual's strong desire to compete and to become Number One. In addition, most writers have discussed how the Type A person is infatuated with "right now," he is under enormous time pressure as he drinks his instant coffee, instant breakfast, while listening to the instant news over headphone radio.

Redford Williams (1993) in his article "Hostility and the Heart" pointed out that of the three most common characteristics of the Type A personality—hurriedness, competitiveness, and hostility—hostility has the least redeeming social or psychological value and was the major toxic component in Type A behavior. In his research, Williams found that those who scored high on a fifty-item questionnaire designed to assess hostility were more afflicted with severe coronary blockages than other patients. Furthermore, he found that more than 70 percent of patients with high scores had severe blockages. In contrast, fewer than 50 percent of those with low hostility scores had a marked blockage of any coronary artery. He also learned that merely recalling an incident which made a subject angry could lead to a deterioration in the heart's pumping efficiency.

The fact that hostile individuals have higher-than-normal increases in blood pressure and stress hormones when they are feeling hostile suggests that they have a low threshold for triggering the sympathetic nervous system's "fight or flight" stress response (see Chapter 1). In addition, hostile people are slower than others to activate the parasympathetic nervous system, the part that can protect the body from the onslaught of stress hormones (Williams 1989, 1993).

Social Support

Virtually every researcher who has related to the stress component in heart disease has commented on the lack of social support in the life of the heart disease victim. What has not been completely understood as yet is the relationship between the individual's hostility and his or her lack of close interpersonal relationships. My own clinical and personal experience has led me to view the relationship as an interactive one. When an individual is mistrustful, frequently angry, and aggressive (all components of Type A behavior), he or she is going to antagonize others and keep alienating them. By the same token, being alienated from relatives, friends, and colleagues can activate and intensify anger.

Flannery (1990) has cited such empirical evidence showing that disruption in human attachments is linked to heart disease and premature death. A major researcher in this area is James Lynch (1977, 1985), who has identified how the presence of caring others may lead to cardiovascular benefits. The presence of caring others seems to stabilize and strengthen heart rate and stabilize and lower blood pressure. Conversely, harmful human attachments appear to lead to cardiovascular dysfunctions. Lynch has shown that for both sexes, for all ages, and for all races, the unmarried (who are frequently lonely) have a higher rate of premature death from heart disease. This is true even if the individual is young. Married women between the ages of 25 and 30 who are widowed have at least a two times greater chance of heart disease than married women of the same age.

Dean Ornish (1990), as part of his program in reversing heart disease, arranges for every patient to be part of a weekly support group where feelings are shared and emotional intimacy is encouraged. Says Ornish:

> Over time, I began to realize that the group support itself was one of the most powerful interventions, as it addressed what I am beginning to believe is a more fundamental cause of why we feel stressed and, in turn, why we get illnesses like heart disease: the perception of isolation.
>
> In short, anything that promotes a sense of isolation

> leads to chronic stress and, often, to illnesses like
> heart disease. Conversely, anything that leads to real
> intimacy and feelings of connection can be healing
> in the real sense of the word: to bring together, to
> make whole. The ability to be intimate has long
> been seen as a key to emotional health; I believe it is
> essential to the health of our hearts as well. [p. 97]

One of the major etiological factors in social isolation, which will be discussed further in later chapters, is that the adult as a child often felt isolated and not well understood by parents and siblings. His or her inevitable anger often repeats itself with peers. Social isolation seems to begin in early childhood and continues indefinitely throughout adult years.

What has not received sufficient attention in the literature on social isolation and its accompanying hostility is how all of us tend to recapitulate destructive relationships from the past in the present. Many adults unconsciously seek out marital partners who remind them of parents and then argue and fight with their spouses in order to discharge resentment toward parental figures (Strean 1980, 1985). The unresolved hostility from the past can also be expressed in work relationships and elsewhere. What needs to be understood by the helping practitioner is that the Type A person who is angry and socially isolated *wants* to hate. He or she derives unconscious gratification from sustaining problematic, destructive relationships (Strean 1995a). Until he or she faces his or her wish to fight, only limited reversal of heart disease can take place. Consequently, helping practitioners must keep this constantly in mind as they work with heart disease patients and their families.

Strengths and Limitations of the Type A Formulation

Friedman and Rosenman's (1981, 1984) conceptualization of the Type A personality was a major step forward in showing that the body and mind truly interact. By identifying Type A individuals for us and showing that they are habitually driven, competitive, and egocentric, we can appreciate the fact that they are going to be under a great deal of stress and therefore prone to heart disease. The formulation provides assistance to both physicians and mental health professionals in knowing just what type of personality is likely to be a heart disease victim. Further, as the heart disease victim comes alive in flesh and blood, those who help him or her professionally can more easily feel empathy toward a real person with real characteristics. In short, the Type A formulation reduces some of the vagueness of the mind–body relationship; a person with specific personality characteristics and with a heart condition comes into sharper focus.

Although the Type A formulation is descriptive, it has almost no explanatory power. It does not answer questions such as: Why is the patient so driven? How do we account for his or her unresolved hostility, cynicism, intense need for advancement and recognition? What childhood experiences contribute to the formation of his or her personality? What types of relationships does he or she form as an adult? What type of healing relationships does this person need? These questions have not really been considered in sufficient depth by professionals working with heart disease patients and they are, of course, the main consideration of this book.

The Stress–Resistant Personality

Just as there are individuals such as the Type A personality who are constantly experiencing stress, there are those who seem to be able to avoid it. Who are these people?

Raymond Flannery (1990), in his book *Becoming Stress-Resistant*, has discussed the characteristics of stress-resistant persons:

1. *Personal control.* Flannery's research found that those who were stress-resistant attempted to exercise reasonable control of stressful situations rather than rely on others. They were self-initiated, self-directed people.
2. *Task-involvement.* People who were stress-resistant were involved in tasks to which they were very committed. The commitment could be to families, careers, community projects, or hobbies.
3. *Lifestyle choices.* Certain patterns of daily behavior employed by stress-resistant persons have been helpful in reducing stress. These include a reduction in caffeine and nicotine and an increase in both aerobic exercise and relaxation procedures. Flannery points out that caffeine and nicotine can increase stress in the body even when no problems are present.
4. *Social support.* Stress-resistant people, as Lynch (1977, 1985) has pointed out, receive a great deal of social support and have many mutually caring attachments.
5. *Humor.* Stress-resistant people often try to see the paradoxes in life and do not always take life too seriously.

us values. Stress-resistant people abide by
values such as the Golden Rule. Many of them
ive in churches and synagogues.

It is of interest that Flannery's (1990) description of the
stress-resistant person has certain similarities to the Type A
person (Friedman and Rosenman 1981, 1984). Type A behavior, it will be recalled, is characterized by a need for control
and an involvement in tasks. Perhaps Flannery is referring to
a relaxed involvement in tasks and a nondriven need for
control. This would be in contrast to the compulsive need for
control and the over-investment in tasks which are observed
in the Type A personality.

The issue of control obviously needs more careful research. Perhaps one of the variables is how the individual
experiences control. Angier (1995), in the article "How
Biology Affects Behavior and Vice Versa," points to studies
in stress research in which scientists have sought to understand what distinguishes a person subject to much stress from
one who is not. They have found that an essential factor is a
matter of the subject's opinion—whether or not the person
believes he or she is in control of a situation. The individual
may or may not actually be in control but simply feeling so
profoundly affects one's circulatory system.

Angier (1995) has discussed the Type B person who is the
opposite of the Type A individual. Type B people are described as self-assured, self-motivated, unrushed, and good
planners. They do not compete too much nor do they compulsively display their achievements. They find confidence in self-approval. Just as Type A behavior has a number of harmful
physiological effects such as increased blood pressure and
heart rate, "Type B behavior can help to slow metabolism and

is better for the health of your body" (p. 156).

Similar to Flannery's (1990) perspective, Cortis (1995) believes Type B behavior can be easily learned. Both of these writers tend to underestimate the degree of resistance that exists in all individuals when these individuals attempt to modify attitudes and behavior. Often, changing a *modus vivendi* requires intensive psychotherapeutic assistance.

Managing Stress

Now that it has been confirmed repeatedly that individuals who are under stress have higher blood pressure and are more prone to heart disease, a number of practitioners and researchers have introduced many different stress management procedures. In this section we will briefly review some of these procedures.

One of the pioneers in stress management is the cardiologist Herbert Benson (1976, 1984, 1987, 1993), who in the 1970s introduced "The Relaxation Response." Benson has spent the past two decades conducting pioneering research on the beneficial effects of meditation. He has demonstrated that meditation can lower blood pressure, decrease premature heartbeats, and produce other beneficial effects such as a precipitous drop in the amount in the bloodstream of a chemical called lactate. High levels of lactate have been associated with anxiety and disquietude, low levels with peace and tranquility (Benson 1993). Benson's work suggests that the relaxation response will be useful in diminishing the pathological processes that are caused or made worse by stress.

Meditation, which is an essential part of the relaxation

response, derives from yoga. Yoga is a very powerful system of stress management and includes breathing techniques, visualization, progressive relaxation practices, and self-analysis. These procedures are designed to increase self-awareness and diminish social isolation. The major thesis of yoga is that body and mind function most efficiently and effectively when one is relaxed. When this occurs, performance is enhanced and intimacy is more easily achieved (Ornish 1990).

The modern use of therapeutic imagery usually entails a 20- to 25-minute session that begins with a relaxation exercise to help focus attention and "center" the mind. During a typical session of imagery, the individual focuses on a predetermined image designed to help him or her control a particular symptom ("active imagery") or one allows the mind to conjure up images that give insight into a particular problem ("receptive imagery"). Imagery helps illuminate the connections between stressful circumstances and physical symptoms, where such connections exist. It does this by helping the person to see "the big picture" (Rossman 1993). The following are healing images suggested to heart patients:

1. Your heart is beating regularly.
2. The arteries are dilating and allowing more blood to flow.
3. The blood is flowing smoothly and unobstructed.

Deep breathing is one of the simplest yet most effective stress management techniques. It works both to prevent harmful reactions to stress and to help relieve them. Research (Ornish 1990) has indicated that by practicing deep breathing for a few minutes each day, stressful events become less upsetting.

As we have already discussed briefly in Chapter 1, regular exercise, particularly aerobic exercise, can act as a buffer against stress and may thus help protect the cardiovascular and immune systems from the consequences of stressful events. Frequent exercise seems to reduce anxiety and, according to some research (Sacks 1993), it can help reduce depression.

Strengths and Limitations of Stress Management Procedures

Stress management techniques have many advantages. They assist in the process of relaxation, which in turn lowers heart beat, reduces blood pressure, and lowers cholesterol count. By learning to relax through daily exercises, most individuals are able to bring a relaxed attitude to their total daily living, thus keeping stress at a minimum. With stress minimized, heart disease can begin to be reversed.

What stress management techniques do not do sufficiently is individualize the person and help him or her resolve those situations which are producing stress. For example, stress management techniques do little to modify a conflicted marriage, an explosive parent-child interaction, or other forms of dysfunctional behavior. Phobias, compulsions, and other neurotic behavior are not addressed.

It would appear that for many individuals, psychotherapy, group therapy, or group support is necessary to diminish the stress they are under. In one of these modalities, their unique conflicts will be addressed and they will have the opportunity

to understand how and why their unique histories are recapitulated in the present. Their sense of isolation is reduced as
they see how they relate to the therapist or group members.
They learn how to resolve the resistances which interfere with
their becoming loving and intimate.

In the next chapter we will further discuss some of the
above issues as we examine the cardiac personality and review
some of the therapeutic principles which may be helpful for
him or her.

3

The Cardiac
Personality

Patients with heart problems and those individuals who are candidates for them may be helped to reverse cardiovascular disease if their personality dynamics are understood in greater depth and breadth by helping professionals. In this chapter our aims are twofold:

1. We want to identify the major personality characteristics and conflicts of what we will term "the cardiac personality," and
2. We will discuss some of the important therapeutic principles involved in helping the cardiac personality resolve some of his or her psychological problems.

In the prologue we suggested that by examining the Type A personality more intensively and taking note of when and why this individual has a tendency to cope with stress somatically, the notion of the cardiac personality will evolve with more clarity.

Previously we posed several questions which needed to be answered about the Type A personality. Some of them were: What makes this person so driven, hostile, and competitive? Why does this individual always clamor for recognition and advancement? Why does he or she become so easily and frequently hurt by people and events?

If we take a closer look at Type A behavior, we observe a major theme consistently running throughout it. Type A individuals are chronically dissatisfied; they always want more and want it immediately. Thus, they are constantly driven, excessively competitive, very impatient, and often are workaholics. But why are they so insatiable?

Omnipotence

One way to try to explain the incessant hunger for power and attention that Type A personalities seek is to note the similarity of their behavior to that of an infant. Babies have been likened to "His Majesty the Prince" and "Her Majesty the Princess" because of their strong narcissism and intense quest for omnipotence (Freud 1914). They want what they want when they want it. And, just as the infant has a low frustration tolerance and is very impatient, the Type A personality behaves the same way. Kernberg (1967), in discussing narcissistic patients, really describes several characteristics of both the infant and the Type A personality: "[They have] an unusual degree of self-reference in their interactions with other people, a great need to be loved and admired by others, and a curious apparent contradiction between a very inflated concept of themselves, and an inordinate need for tribute from others" (p. 655). Such patients have also been "characterized by a sense of entitlement and fantasies of omniscience, omnipotence, and perfection of the self" (Moore and Fine 1990, p. 124).

Although all infants appear to be grandiose princes and princesses, with appropriate doses of tender love and care, and timely weaning and other controls, they usually move toward more involvement with the concerns of others and less preoccupation with themselves. However, if they have been traumatized, rejected, excessively indulged, or arbitrarily frustrated, infants can remain fixated at this early level of development and constantly seek to fulfill grandiose desires.

What is important to understand about Type A personalities is that their omnipotent fantasies are strong because of the failure of competent interactions with others early in life. As adults they feel forced to turn to omnipotent solutions because the realities of life are too difficult for them to face (J. Novick and K. Novick 1991). Type A personalities find reality so tough to take because if they are not treated like royalty, they experience themselves as weak paupers who have no standing at all with others. If they are not "machos" they feel like weaklings. If they don't hit the equivalent of home runs, then they are "strike out queens." In effect, if they are not the best, they are the worst.

Although we will examine the early histories of Type A personalities in subsequent chapters, what may be said now is that these individuals have to resort to omnipotent behavior because early in their development they were made to feel like "nobodies." Feeling displaced by the arrival of siblings, demeaned by one or both parents, feeling disfavored and humiliated by family members and others, Type A personalities are desperately trying to prove to themselves that they are somebody rather than nobody.

J. Novick and K. Novick (1991) have pointed out that the picture clinicians usually portray in describing omnipotent fantasies of adult patients "is of a raging, hostile tyrant whose behavior is fueled by envy and compensates for feelings of helplessness and shame" (p. 310). Similarly, Kernberg (1988) has noted that there is a curious discrepancy between the state of omnipotence attributed to the infant and the adult. The happy, contented infant, safe in mother's arms, is said to be in a state of infantile omnipotence, a happy delusion that he or she is the center of the universe with the power to make everyone meet all of his or her needs. But when we discuss fantasies of omnipotence in adults, we are not referring to blissful daydreams, rather we are alluding to hostile fantasies of complete control over others. Chassegut-Smiegel (1984) described omnipotent fantasies in adults as *the murder of reality*.

Under the impact of extreme and frequent disappointment, Type A personalities as children turned away from their inborn capacities to interact effectively with the real world and began to use their rage and pain to control others. The failure of reality-oriented competence to effect empathic attunement (Kohut 1977) forced the child "into an imaginary world where safety, attachment, and omnipotent control were magically associated with pain" (J. Novick and K. Novick 1991, p. 313).

Joyce McDougall (1985), who has done much research and therapeutic work with Type A individuals, describes them as *striving for the impossible*. She notes that this phenomenon is an omnipotent attempt to control other people's thoughts and actions, to deny the undeniable, to reconcile the irreconcilable, to destroy and yet retain the other person, to die and yet live forever. She has also suggested that to help someone accept the impossibility of gratifying omnipotent fantasies is a most difficult task.

There seems to be a direct relationship between omnipotent fantasies and health habits. Many Type A individuals feel they can completely control the world around them, including their own bodies. So they say, "Who needs salads, cholesterol readings, or doctors?" Many Type A personalities take better care of their cars than they do of their own bodies (Schardt 1995).

When children are forced through experiences such as weaning and toilet training to renounce their belief in their omnipotence, they turn to adults around them, who they believe are omnipotent. Through introjection and identification children try to restore their own omnipotence. Certain narcissistic feelings of well-being are characterized by the fact that they are felt as a reunion with an omnipotent force (Fenichel 1945). This accounts for the Type A personality's propensity to seek admiration and adulation. Through the praise and recognition he or she receives, a paradise that was lost seems to be regained temporarily.

One of the difficult problems for individuals who have omnipotent fantasies is that they are always being frustrated and insulted. Because they want the world to cater to them constantly, gratify them consistently, and always treat them as majesty, the world becomes a dreadful and depriving place. This accounts for the Type A personality's strong competitiveness—he or she must be Number One and anything less is disastrous.

Obviously, when a king or queen is knocked off the throne constantly, anger erupts.

Hostility

Having reviewed the strong omnipotent fantasies of Type A individuals, we are now in a better position to appreciate why they are so frequently and intensely hostile. Although these individuals are always striving to control their surroundings, most of the time their wishes are being thwarted. When they cannot drive their cars at the speed they want, but must be in a traffic jam with others, they feel insulted and humiliated as if they were deprived and misunderstood children. To cope with their dreadful loss, they attack others. The waiter who keeps them waiting feels to them like an inattentive and unloving mother who should be rebuked. The boss or the employee who does not smile may remind them of family members who were demeaning, and thus the employee must be castigated. Anybody or anything that robs the throne from the Type A individual is experienced as a cruel, tyrannical force and must be hurt. Eventually, almost everybody and everything becomes an enemy.

As discussed in Chapter 1, we live in a "hate culture" (Fine 1990) where most individuals are trying to outdo others and become Number One. Competition in our culture is more valued than cooperation, and achievement is ascribed high value, particularly social and economic achievements. Consequently, hatred has become a way of life in many sectors of our society and has invaded many dimensions of family life. As a result, we have more Type A personalities in our society than any other personality type. Hence, if the Type A personality is most prone to heart disease, it would follow that in our society heart disease would be the number one killer, as it is.

Our culture is so filled with hatred that human destructiveness is often taken for granted and becomes a fact of life. Two well known psychiatrists, Richard C. Friedman and Jennifer Downey (1995) state:

> There has never been a time in all recorded history without war and violent crime. Our species appears to have an omnivorous appetite for destruction. We are the "natural enemies" of each other, of most other mammalian species, including those who have no other natural enemies, and even of other diverse life forms that constitute the planetary ecosystem. [p. 253]

E. Wilson (1978), in his book *On Human Nature*, has written:

> Human aggression cannot be explained as either a dark angelic flaw or a bestial instinct. Nor is it the pathological symptom of upbringing in a cruel environment. Human beings are strongly predisposed to respond with unreasoning hatred to external threats and to escalate their hostility sufficiently to overwhelm the source of the threat by a respectably wide margin of safety. Our brains do appear to be programmed to the following extent: we are inclined to partition other people into friends and aliens. In the same sense that birds are inclined to learn territorial songs and to navigate by the polar constellations, we tend to fear deeply the actions of strangers and to solve conflict by aggression. These roles are most likely to have evolved during the past hundreds of thousands of years of human evolution and thus have conferred a biological advantage on those who have conformed to them with the greatest fidelity. [p.119]

What is frequently overlooked in assessing the hostility of Type A personalities is the tremendous frustration of pleasure needs they endured early in life. This pain of frustration and the resulting hatred gradually form a wall, a barrier within an individual, so that friendship and joy are rarely achieved. This same frustration and resulting hatred build up to form pessimism, depression of spirits, indifference, and even oppression of others (English and Pearson 1945). The "cynicism" of the Type A personality which Friedman and Rosenman (1981, 1984) have referred to is really a wall of pessimism and depression which is part of a hostile view of the world.

One of the most obvious goals of the hostile person is to hurt others frequently in order to humiliate them. But it is important to remember that Type A individuals wish to hurt others because they have been hurt. In effect, they do to others what has been done to them. In Anna Freud's (1946) terms, they "identify with the aggressor." As they identify with the aggressor, they appear like those children who have experienced much pain, anguish, and humiliation in having their tonsils taken out. What do these children do in order to act out their revenge? They get a toy stethoscope, become a doctor in their fantasy, and in their play brutally take out the tonsils of everybody in sight.

Coping with Hostility: The Type A Way

Although some individuals, on occasion, can discharge hostility and feel better, this is not the case for most of us. When we attack others directly or in fantasy, we usually feel quite anxious. The anxiety is caused by two factors:

1. When we attack someone, we invariably expect retaliation and often of a more severe kind than the

blow we dealt, and

2. Most of the time when we attack, we feel remorseful afterwards because we fear the loss of love, admiration, and respect that we want from the one we attacked.

Because they are so desirous of love, admiration, and respect, Type A personalities are constantly feeling threatened by even feeling hostility, let alone expressing it. To lose love is one of their greatest sources of stress. And, because they know they are frequently harboring hostility, they are almost always experiencing enormous agitation lest the hostility be revealed to those whose love and admiration they so desperately seek.

It is the turmoil and agitation accruing from undischarged hostility that eventually affects the workings of the heart and promotes heart disease (Cannon 1963, Charash 1991, Chopra 1993, Cortis 1995, Ornish 1990). The intense struggle that Type A personalities have with rage may very well be one of the leading contributors to their heart disease (Schneider 1967).

Inasmuch as the individuals we are discussing are constantly on the warpath in their fantasy life, they eventually become quite paranoid. Simmering with hostility which frightens them, they are always ready for retaliation. Although most clinicians refer to the Type A personality's "cynicism" and "distrust," this description tends to be too mild. Careful listening to Type A personalities' remarks and careful observation of their actions reveals a paranoid view of the world. Their employees are "out to get" them. Frequently their spouses and children are "trying to take control away" from them, and their colleagues are continually "gossiping" about them. Eventually the whole world becomes "a rotten place" and indeed, paranoia reigns!

In contrast to sociopaths who can hurt others and are not incessantly preoccupied about the effects of their attacks, the individuals we are describing have a strict conscience or superego (Alexander 1965). Thus, they are constantly feeling strong pangs of guilt. Convinced that they should be punished, they become very masochistic.

Those physicians and mental health workers who have worked with patients suffering from heart disease and other Type A personalities have commented on their inability to enjoy pleasure. These people are workaholics and chronic worriers (Cortis 1995, Cousins 1983). Attempts to get them to enjoy themselves are futile until they can be helped to get in touch with their guilt and need for punishment. They feel constantly remorseful because they are very upset about their murderous wishes which are rarely discussed by them (Reik 1941).

When hostility cannot be handled well, as is true of the Type A personality, the individual regresses and wants to be taken care of. However, his or her dependency wishes cause conflict as well.

Dependency Conflicts

With omnipotent desires thwarted and strong hostile fantasies causing much guilt, Type A personalities don't know which way to turn for comfort, and then they begin to feel helpless. This helplessness inevitably stirs up strong yearnings to be nurtured and even indulged. However, Type A personalities strongly defend against their dependency wishes and try instead to appear autonomous and self-reliant. They view depending on others as a sign of weakness.

One way that many Type A personalities cope with their passive-dependent yearnings is by turning to nonhuman objects for gratification. As anyone who has visited a cardiac rehabilitation unit will attest, many of the patients are obese. Food becomes a source of love and comfort for many of them as they repudiate contact with human beings. Coffee can serve as the equivalent of mother's milk and alcohol can provide the lift that is lacking in their interpersonal relationships. A smoking addiction can be a substitute for a love affair. May (1991) has noted that patients who have become addicted have turned alcohol, food, or drugs into fantasied individuals and have a "transference" relationship toward them. Food or drugs are related to as if they were parents, siblings, or lovers who can give them comfort and pleasure.

Since food, tobacco, alcohol, or drugs are poor substitutes for interpersonal gratification, the Type A personality becomes a very lonely and isolated person. Virtually every researcher who has discussed the psychological components of heart disease refers to the patients' enormous sense of isolation (for example, Chopra 1993, Cortis 1995, Cousins 1983, Ornish 1990). It is not that these men and women do not have friends and acquaintances; often they have an active social life. What accounts for their loneliness is that they cannot allow themselves to feel dependent on others in an intimate way. They can be friendly, but not loving; talkative, but not spontaneous.

Schneider (1967) has averred that those individuals who have heart attacks are literally suffering from "a broken heart." They feel very rejected by someone whose love they have craved but they cannot allow themselves to know how desperate and needy they really feel; it is too humiliating for them to acknowledge the truth. These are also the sentiments of Lynch (1977), who, in his book *The Broken Heart: The Medical Consequences of Loneliness,* has presented much empirical data demonstrating the strong link between social isolation and heart disease.

Although many writers have recognized the normal place of dependence in human existence (for example, Moore and Fine 1990, Parens and Saul 1971), dependency usually carries a pejorative meaning, implying the need to lean on others in an excessive and age-inappropriate way. Though there are cultural taboos placed on dependency wishes in our society, many individuals fail to recognize that all human interaction requires some form of dependency. The reason that pejorative meanings are often assigned to dependency is because depending on another person often stimulates wishes to regress and become a child. This is repugnant to many, particularly the Type A personality who, as we have stressed, must appear independent at all times.

Dependency is frequently associated with orality (Freud 1905a) because the infant's earliest feelings of pleasure originate in this area. If the infant's oral desires have been gratified, he or she becomes a trusting individual (Erikson 1950), if not, the infant becomes a distrustful and pessimistic person, two characteristics of the Type A personality (Moore and Fine 1990).

A Psychosomatic Solution

When an individual has grandiose fantasies which are always being frustrated, reactive hostility which cannot be expressed, and regression to a position of infantile dependency which cannot be acknowledged, then the body takes over. As discussed in Chapters 1 and 2, when individuals cannot put into words what they feel and think, they use their bodies to express their conflicts.

When the body is used to express conflicts, why is the heart unconsciously "chosen" to communicate distress? The men and women that we have been discussing have "put their hearts" into efforts to be the equivalent of kings and queens. Admiration, love, and control of their universe are "heartily" sought. When these valuable psychic commodities are not available in the quantities desired, these individuals first are furious but follow this up by becoming masochistic or "heartsick." Feeling dependent wishes, they become frightened of them and must deny their desires, and they become "heartbroken" instead. As we stated earlier (Schneider 1967), research has demonstrated that many individuals who suffer heart attacks have felt abandoned or rejected by an important love object. This was certainly evident in the vignettes we discussed at the beginning of Chapter 2 and in the prologue as well.

The Cardiac Personality

When Type A personalties cannot cope with their omnipotence, hostility, and dependency, and cannot put their feelings, thoughts, and memories into words, they often become victims of heart disease. We are designating these individuals *cardiac personalities*. They can be described as Type A personalities, that is, driven, competitive, hostile, and cynical. But, on closer examination, they are really deeply frustrated children who are desperate about their loss of power, furious because they cannot regain it, lonely and dependent because they are so mistrustful, inarticulate because they are embarrassed by their thoughts and feelings, and tend to become physically sick with heart disease because they cannot cope with their psychological conflicts.

Joyce McDougall (1989) has described how Type A individuals become heart patients, that is, cardiac personalities. A summary of her findings follows:

> 1. Certain cardiac reactions are a somatic expression of an attempt to protect oneself against narcissistic longings which are felt to be life-endangering, much as a small infant might experience the threat of death.

> 2. To achieve this purpose, the psyche in moments of danger sends, as in infancy, a primitive psychic message of warning to the body which bypasses the use of language. Therefore the danger cannot be thought about.

> 3. The psychic message might result in heightened blood pressure, quickened pulse rate, or other heart dysfunctions.

> 4. The emotion aroused is not recognized in a symbolic way, that is, within the code of language which would have allowed the affect-laden representations to be named, thought about, and dealt with by the mind, but instead is immediately transmitted by the mind to the body. This is done in a primitive, nonverbal way such as flight-fight impulses, and produces the physical disorganization that we call a psychosomatic symptom.

5. The physical suffering the heart disease causes is liable to be compensated by the conviction that the disease is serving a protective function.

6. Communicating a state of despair through the illness may be the only way to gain access to caretaking people. [pp. 28-29]

Eysenck (1991), who has also researched the cardiac personality extensively, concluded that the major etiological factor in heart disease is "suppression of emotion." Although Eysenck does not specify which emotions are suppressed, his reports seem to suggest that his subjects were suffering from the triad which we have been discussing in this chapter—frustrated omnipotence, repressed hostility, and unresolved dependency problems (Grossarth-Maticek and H. Eysenck 1990).

Cameron (1963) has also focused on "the cardiac personality" without labelling the individual with heart disease as such. In his discussion of some of the psychological factors involved in heart disease, he states that the heart condition "puts an apparent or an actual physical illness in place of an intolerable current situation. [It causes] a person to be physically sick instead of becoming neurotic or psychotic" (p. 685). He further points out that although heart disease "often involves primary anxiety—the diffuse, regressive anxiety of a small child—this may be easier to bear than a secondary anxiety based upon conscious conflicts over childhood impulses, which a person cannot otherwise control and does not recognize" (p. 685). As other authors also have pointed out (for example, McDougall 1985, Scherwitz et al. 1978), Cameron (1963) suggests that heart disease gives these patients the privileges of a sick person without interfering with their freedom or lowering their self esteem.

> The secondary gain, as this is called, and the relationship of an unconsciously needed dependency upon a parent-figure, the clinician, can bring valuable gratification to a basically immature person. These gratifications should not be scorned. They sometimes protect a person from disabling neurotic or psychotic developments, and they often give meaningful interpersonal relationships to an otherwise empty life. It should be added that many emotionally immature dependent men and women hide their needs, from themselves as well as from others, being an energetic, independent, facade. The needs are still there, however, and they are still unsatisfied.

> Finally, there remains to be considered the intensification of [heart disease] by a psychosomatic disorder. The patient may use his physical illness as a means of eliciting concern, care and affection, which he has needed all along, but has been unable to get as long as he remained well. This also should not be scorned. Life is objectively more difficult and less rewarding for some persons than for others, and subjectively it may seem bleak, even though objectively it is considered fortunate. [p. 686]

Some Strengths of the Cardiac Personality

There is a tendency among mental health and other professionals to focus too exclusively on neurotic and other dysfunctional behavior and neglect considering their patients' adaptive strengths. By doing this, they fail to individualize their patients, and therefore cannot fully resolve diagnostic and prognostic issues nor arrange for their patients to receive a treatment plan specifically designed for them. It should be mentioned parenthetically that there is much variation in the population of cardiac personalities. Not only are there differences among them with regard to the intensity and pervasiveness of their conflicts around omnipotence, hostility, and dependency, but there is also variation among them regarding their personality assets.

While always keeping individual differences in mind, it is helpful to review some of the ego strengths that are quite common among cardiac personalities. In my many interviews and other contacts with cardiac patients, including my participation in the support group in which I have been a patient, I have never met a cardiac personality who did not have a keen sense of humor. This is quite consistent with what we know both about the psychodynamics of cardiac personalities and the psychology of humor (Freud 1905b, Strean 1993b).

One of the major gratifications in listening to and telling jokes and/or involving ourselves in other forms of humorous interaction is that forbidden impulses are discharged in fantasy. Cardiac personalities often experience their own hostility as unacceptable to them. Therefore, jokes and anecdotes which provide an opportunity to discharge aggression vicariously and which cannot be expressed in daily life are very appealing to cardiac personalities. In addition, when cardiac personalities get a good laugh in response to their humor, they not only receive permission to secretly discharge their latent animosity, but they receive the love and adulation they are seeking.

Warren Poland (1994), in "The Gift of Laughter: On the Development of a Sense of Humor in Clinical Analysis," stated: "The facilitating of the development of the patient's capacity for mature humor is one of the happiest and proudest effects of clinical analysis" (p. 23). He also suggested that humor provides an opportunity for sustenance and consolation throughout life. It offers self-comfort without complete denial.

In addition to possessing a sense of humor, many cardiac personalities are intelligent individuals, very interested in the world around them. Their intellectual curiosity often propels them to learn more about their heart disease and about themselves as individuals. In cardiac rehabilitation centers across the country, many of the patients are "experts" on heart disease, very knowledgeable about stress, and keenly aware of the psychodynamics of the cardiac personality (Cortis 1995).

Because of their severe superego commands, cardiac personalities are generally law abiding, cooperative individuals. Although they have strong wishes to rebel, as we have already discussed, they place severe restraints on their tendencies to aggress. In addition, their desire to achieve, excel, and accomplish is an asset in group and individual psychotherapy, as it is in exercising, obeying dietary rules, and in stress management.

In spite of cardiac personalities not easily asking for help—their omnipotent wishes interfere—they can allow themselves to participate in therapeutic programs that are designed to help their hearts. This is less threatening than asking for help with their psyches, which is difficult for them to do. Thus, when they are told that it will help their heart condition to talk about their feelings, many cardiac personalities have an interest in meeting with a therapist. Those who have worked with cardiac patients often have heard the sentiment, "If it helps my heart, I'll talk about myself." This statement seems to protect the individual against feelings of vulnerability and tends to deny any dependency gratification.

Some Therapeutic Principles for Treating Cardiac Personalities

The therapeutic principles that we will discuss in this section are applicable to other patients in need of psychological help, but they are here designed specifically for the cardiac personality. Keeping in mind the conflicts of the cardiac personality that we have been discussing in this chapter, the therapeutic interventions reviewed in this section are aimed to assist helping professionals—physicians, nurses, exercise physiologists, dieticians, and mental health professionals—to use themselves in ways that will help cardiac patients reduce their stress and increase their capacities to enjoy life, like themselves more, and love others more deeply and consistently.

Making a Referral for Psychotherapeutic Help

Helping a cardiac personality to accept the idea of talking to an expert about his or her feelings and conflicts is rarely an easy task. The very nature of psychotherapeutic help involves sharing vulnerabilities and acknowledging limitations and conflicts. Being placed in this position runs contrary to the cardiac personalities' strong wish for control and one-upmanship. Further, the idea of depending on someone who knows more and has special skills often feels offensive.

Anybody who wants to refer a cardiac personality for therapeutic help has to be ready to hear all kinds of resistive statements, including hostile and demeaning statements toward the one who is trying to make the referral. The last thing the person making the referral wants to do is argue about the merits of psychotherapy. It only compounds the prospective patient's reluctance to receive help. Rather, the referring individual not only has to make the suggestion tactfully but also has to be very understanding and empathetic when rebuffed.

> When Arthur, a man in his fifties asked his cardiologist what he could do to help diminish the intensity of his heart problems, his physician recommended increased exercise, changes in his diet, and talking to an expert such as a psychologist. Arthur had no problem accepting the exercise and diet recommendations, but with regard to the psychotherapy, he stated, "I'm not going to expose myself to somebody who wants me to be a kid and talk about my childhood. I'm not that weak or dependent."

> The cardiologist, sensitive to Arthur's resistances and empathizing with his concern, said, "I certainly don't want to encourage you to do something which you abhor." Seeing that the cardiologist was not going to try to control or pressure him, Arthur became more interested and less opposed to psychotherapy. He asked, "If I don't like it, am I committed to this procedure for a long time?" The cardiologist suggested, "I don't think you should commit yourself to

any procedure you question. You can try it out and then quit."

A week later, Arthur requested the name and phone number of a therapist and followed this up by arranging for a series of interviews.

Many times a suggestion to an individual that he or she might consider psychotherapy needs not one but many discussions. The person making the referral should never be in a rush to complete the process, otherwise the effort will backfire.

> When Bertha, a woman in her mid-fifties, was advised by a nutritionist that her heart problems and obesity were due to stress, she seemed quite interested in discussing the nutritionist's ideas further. But when Bertha was told that she should consider having counseling immediately and that the nutritionist had a person for her to see and could arrange an appointment for the next day, Bertha felt overwhelmed and abruptly ended the interview.

> It took Bertha another 6 months of talking to various professionals before she would even consider having a consultation with a therapist.

In sum, suggesting to a cardiac personality that he or she should consider receiving counseling or psychotherapy is usually a complex and difficult task. It requires careful timing, enormous tact, and considerable patience. The individual making the referral should not expect the candidate for therapy to accept the matter immediately. It is usually greeted with considerable ambivalence and resistance. The candidate for therapy needs much time to discuss doubts and uncertainties and have his or her resistances thoroughly respected.

The Crucial Importance of Listening

When the cardiac personality (or any other person experiencing stress) dares to share problems with a relative or friend, most of the time he or she is greeted with advice, reassurance, quick judgments, and reminiscences of the listener.

One of the most curative dimensions of counseling and psychotherapy, particularly for the cardiac personality, is to have someone listen empathetically without saying very much. Many helping professionals underestimate the value of patient listening and overestimate the value of their interpretations and other verbalizations.

Cardiac personalities, as we have already indicated, have not received sufficient individualized attention during their childhood and adolescent years. Often, they have been the victims of authoritarian attitudes and pressuring commands. Of more importance, they have had limited opportunity to talk about their feelings—their hurt, anger, doubts, and vulnerabilities—without having their views censored or devalued. Consequently, perhaps even more than most patients in psychotherapy, cardiac personalities very much welcome uninterrupted listening from the helping professional.

Patients begin to value themselves much more when they feel their therapists value what they say. This can only take place if the recipient of psychotherapy has as a therapist a quiet, nonintrusive, empathetic listener.

Asking Questions

One of the central procedures in good interviewing with the cardiac patient is posing good questions. A question that truly engages the inteviewee is one that clarifies ambiguities, completes a picture of the situation being described, obtains more detail about the patient's thinking, and elicits emotional responses (Kadushin 1972). Cardiac personalities, because they are usually intellectually sophisticated individuals who have many undischarged emotions, easily get bored with routine, mechanical questions. They want to be emotionally engaged and individualized. As we now know, they abhor being one of the crowd.

Questions have to be phrased so that they can be under-stood. They should be unambiguous and simple enough for the interviewee to remember what is being asked. Questions that can be answered with "no" or "yes" do not really help the person to discharge feelings and tensions nor relate facts. If an interviewee is asked, "Do you like your boss?" he or she is given limited opportunity to reflect on attitudes toward the boss. Yet, if the interviewee is asked, "Can you tell me about your boss?" the chances of more data being elicited are enchanced (Strean 1994a).

Above all, the candidate for psychotherapy, to address a question, must feel that it comes from an interested and empathetic questioner. Otherwise, there is little motivation to become involved in the therapy. The cardiac personality is always testing the therapist's motives. His or her distrust and cynicism are forever present. Consequently, questions must emanate from a professional who truly cares and is truly curious.

The Inevitability of Transference

Inasmuch as all of us bring our unique histories, memories, wishes, fears, conscience, and defenses into all relationships, nobody perceives anybody without some distortion. In all interpersonal relationships nonrational, subjective factors are present.

Cardiac personalites, because they are very much influenced by their past experiences and memories, are very likely to distort their therapists and see them as ungiving, critical parents; or, they can idealize them and make them the parents they wished they had.

Transference, although existing in all relationships, can become quite intense in a therapeutic interaction. The nature of psychotherapy involves depending on an expert for understanding and help. Thus, feelings and fears that the patient entertains toward important figures of the past on whom he or she depended will inevitably be transferred to the therapist.

Inasmuch as cardiac personalities are very prone to transference reactions, if clinicians do not understand how they are being experienced by them, they cannot be very helpful. If a patient loves the therapist, the patient will be inclined to accept most of the therapist's interventions. If the patient hates the therapist, even the most neutral question by the therapist will be suspect. Finally, if the patient has mixed feelings toward the therapist, almost all of the therapist's comments and actions will be experienced ambivalently.

Regardless of the setting in which they are being treated, the therapeutic modality used, or the therapist's skills and years of experience, all cardiac personalities (as is true of all patients in therapy and counseling) will respond to interventions in terms of the current transference. It is important for clinicians of all persuasions to recognize that the most brilliant statement in the world by a therapist will be refuted by a patient who is in a negative transference. It is equally important for counselors and therapists to recognize that the most inaccurate statement in the world will be totally accepted if the patient is in a positive transference.

A major task in therapeutic work with cardiac personalities is to help them see how and why they experience the therapist the way they do. Why does one patient argue with the therapist almost every time the latter says something? Why does another patient act like a compliant child and accept almost everything the therapist says? Of course, the therapist has to possess a clear understanding of how the patient experienced significant others in order to help the latter understand and master how transferences influence his or her current functioning.

Although transference reactions are always traceable to childhood, there is not a simple one-to-one correspondence between the past and present. Frequently, cardiac personalites demonstrate what Fine (1982) has called a "compensatory fantasy." This is a fantasy about the therapist that the patient actively entertains and believes in order to make up for what was lacking in childhood. Therefore, the therapist is often pictured as "an ideal parent," "a perfect lover," " a most brilliant teacher," and so forth.

Transference reactions can take many forms. The patient can proclaim loving feelings toward the therapist, but other behavior such as forgetting appointments, coming constantly late to them, or bouncing a check, may reveal the opposite. Similarly, statements of hatred may defend against warm feelings.

A very common use of the transference is the patient's projection onto the therapist of the patient's psychic structure—wishes, defenses, or values. Many therapists are experienced as dirty old men or dirty old women because patients project their own forbidden and unacceptable sexual and aggressive wishes onto the therapist. An even more frequent phenomenon is the patient projecting onto the therapist his or her own superego mandates. This is why patients are frequently anticipating criticism or other forms of punishment from the therapist.

As the therapist and patient accept transference as a fact of therapeutic life and consistently examine the patient's transference responses, they gain an appreciation of the nature of the patient's conflicts and those aspects of the patient's history that are contributing to his or her stress and heart problems.

Transference Reactions of Cardiac Personalities: Some Examples

Idealizing the Therapist

Most individuals, but particularly cardiac personalities, yearn for a perfect parent. In therapy, where the patient, often for the first time in his or her life, finds an empathetic listener who asks for little but gives a great deal, it is not difficult for the patient to believe: "At last, I have found the ideal parent." Then the patient soaks in every word of the therapist, truly believes that Paradise has been discovered, and feels like an overjoyed child.

Although this idealization should be accepted by the therapist and not contradicted, it is important for the therapist to recognize that he or she is being severely distorted; otherwise, the patient will be hurt. The patient will feel that he or she has the right to be a child forever, and therefore will never achieve much self-confidence or self-esteem. He or she will remain a psychological child tied to a parent.

> Charles, a man in his late forties, was referred to a female therapist by his physician because, in addition to his problems with angina, he was quite depressed. Almost as soon as he began therapy, he felt much better and his depression lifted. Having a mother figure giving him attention and empathy satisfied a craving of his that was frustrated early in his childhood. Charles felt that his therapist was the most "nurturing, kindest, attentive woman" he had ever met in his life.

> For some time, therapist and patient enjoyed each other, each soaking in the other's laudatory remarks. The treatment was reminiscent of the initial stages of a love affair, and Charles and his therapist were enthralled with themselves and each other.

> When it became apparent to the therapist, and later to Charles himself, that he was not growing from his therapeutic experience, the therapist began to monitor her exultation when Charles incessantly complimented her. Eventually Charles got in touch with the aggression behind his childish facade and began to observe how frightened he was to assert himself—a major factor in his depression and major contributor to his heart problems.

The Negative Therapeutic Reaction

Anybody who has worked as a psychotherapist has observed that many patients who achieve insight into their problems and accept their therapists' interpretations do not improve. Sigmund Freud (1923) attributed this occurrence to the fact that there was an inner force at work that prevented patients from utilizing their insights. He identified this force as "a superego resistance."

Freud and the many mental health professionals who have followed him have learned that there are many patients who cannot tolerate the idea of feeling better and enjoying a productive life. Almost every time they do feel pleasure, they feel guilty about it. What clinicians since Freud have been able to appreciate is that guilt-ridden patients with punitive superegos are ones who have strong hostile wishes. When these patients succeed at anything, they worry about whom they have destroyed.

As will be recalled from our discussion of cardiac personalities, they are individuals who have strong hostile wishes but usually keep their rage buried. Consequently, they have a tendency to rebel in an indirect manner and take a passive-aggressive approach to life. Cardiac personalities, who usually have punitive superegos and harbor strong hostile fantasies, bring their *modus vivendi* to the therapeutic situation, as all patients do. When they enter therapy, do not improve, and point out that they won't ever get better, they are directing anger toward the therapist and are unconsciously trying to defeat the therapeutic process.

> Doreen, a single woman in her late thirties, entered therapy because her "whole life was a mess." She was "unsuccess-

ful" in her job as a teacher, was a "social misfit" with men, argued with her women friends, was often depressed, and was occasionally suicidal. She was referred to therapy by her trainer at a fitness center after she complained of chest pains, breathing problems, and "other signs of psychosomatic problems."

Although Doreen carefully listened to and seemed to absorb her therapist's interpretations, she would always return to her misery after a few days. Inasmuch as she eventually had to defeat almost everything the therapist said, Doreen had to defeat her therapist's notion that she was trying to defeat her therapist at every turn. Eventually she left therapy, feeling that it had not helped her very much.

Though most cardiac personalities who have negative therapeutic reactions eventually become aware of the futility of their battles with the therapist, there are some like Doreen who derive more satisfaction from fighting than cooperating. What is important for the clinician to keep in mind in working with cardiac personalities is that almost all of them have wishes to oppose and defeat the therapist. Having endured many slings and arrows in their past, and having felt defeated by parents and others on many occasions, they frequently want the therapist to feel defeated. The therapist must always be alert to this eventuality and help the patient to feel safe enough to discharge resentment in the therapy, particularly toward the therapist.

The Erotic Transference

When cardiac patients have found "the ideal person" in the form of a therapist, they can fall in love with the therapist and have many sexual fantasies toward him or her. The erotic transference can have almost any dynamic meaning. As Fine (1982) has commented about the erotic transference:

> It may be a bid for reassurance, a cover-up for hostility, an expression of envy, an oral-incorpora-tive wish, a defense against homosexuality, or all of these at different times.... It is not possible to tell in advance what meaning erotic feelings may have or even to equate different patients merely because they display similar behavior. Each person has to be understood in terms of his or her own background and life experience. [p. 95]

One overlooked dimension of the erotic transference that is often shown by cardiac patients is that the patient is trying to remove the therapist from his or her therapeutic position. Feeling vulnerable and weak in the role of dependent patient, many cardiac personalities experience a sense of power and control, that is, feel omnipotent, when they try to seduce the therapist.

> Eric, a man in his mid-fifties, was referred by his physician for psychotherapy after he showed many symptoms of stress. Eric, who had a mild heart attack in his late forties, suffered from migraine headaches, chronic fatigue, depression, chest pains, and high blood pressure.

> After spending several sessions reviewing his symptom picture and focusing on feelings of depression and vulnera-bility, Eric began to flatter his female therapist. At first he talked about the therapist's kindness and empathy. This was soon followed up with complimentary comments about her clothes and "sexy appearance." Finally, he asked her to go

out with him on a date.

> When the therapist did not censure Eric for wanting to date her, nor agree to go out with him, but encouraged him to discuss his wishes and fantasies, Eric gradually grew impatient and aggressed toward the therapist. He told her she was "too professional," "uptight," and "a coward." Seeing that he could not draw her into combat, Eric slowly acknowledged how uncomfortable he felt as a patient. He talked about feeling weak in most relationships and was eventually able to see how, in most relationships, he was feeling like a weak boy with cold parents.

The erotic transference, like all transference reactions, is an attempt by patients to avoid facing themselves. Cardiac personalities in particular often find it easier to get excited about the therapist than to observe themselves. Eventually, therapists need to help patients confront their resistance to therapy when they manifest an erotic transference.

The Universality of Resistance

Initially most patients enjoy talking about themselves and usually feel better as a result. However, sooner or later the therapy creates anxiety. As patients discover parts of themselves they have hidden, as they confront forbidden fantasies and recover embarrassing memories, they begin to feel guilt and shame. To protect themselves against the uncomfortable feelings of guilt and shame, and to ward off the anxiety that produces it, patients will stop producing material and cease examining themselves. When this happens, we refer to this behavior as resistance.

Resistance is any action or attitude of the patient that impedes the course of therapeutic work. Inasmuch as every patient, to some extent, wants unconsciously to preserve the status quo, all therapy must be carried on in the face of some resistance.

What are referred to as defenses in the patient's daily life, for example, projection, denial, and repression, emerge as resistances in treatment (A. Freud 1946). Defenses are coping mechanisms which we all use to ward off danger. Inasmuch as cardiac personalities almost always feel that danger is around the corner, they are very actively defending themselves and show many resistances in the therapy situation.

> Florence, age 45, a member of a therapy group of men and women who had heart disease, spent most of her time at the group sessions criticizing the other group members. She admonished them for not being firm enough in their daily interactions, criticized them for being too indulgent with their spouses and children, and offered them all kinds of advice in many areas of living.

> When she began to talk about her own marriage, Florence was critical of her husband and told the group that he did not heed her admonitions sufficiently.

> Florence resisted treatment by focusing on everybody's problems except her own. This was exactly how she handled her marital and other interpersonal problems, projecting them onto her husband and others.

Examples of Resistance

In any discussion of resistance, it is important to keep in mind that the specific behavior, such as lateness to an interview, does not tell us very much until we hear more about it from the patient. Lateness can express anything from defiance to a fear of intimacy. Sometimes the specific resistance can express more than one motive.

> George, a man of 55, came for therapy for many reasons. One issue that he wished to explore in treatment was his lack of success in sustaining relationships with women. After falling madly in love, he would abruptly break up with his girlfriends.

> Following about 4 months of treatment with a female therapist, George began coming late for appointments. When his lateness was explored by the therapist, George at first denied that it had "any meaning." However, when the therapist did not challenge his retort, George was able to tell the therapist that he did not want her to feel "too important" or "too dominating" at his expense.

> George's lateness was a symptom of his competition with women and his feeling of vulnerability next to them. As he learned that his competition was related to envious feelings of his younger sister, his lateness diminished and his relationships with women friends improved.

Very often a resistive piece of behavior is an attempt to place the therapist in the same hated position in which the patient was placed in childhood. Inasmuch as cardiac personalities have often felt scapegoated in their original families, they have a strong tendency to scapegoat others. The therapist is often selected as a formidable scapegoat.

> Hillary, a woman in her forties who came into treatment when she found herself in constant arguments with superiors

at her job, began to arrive late for her therapy in the fourth month of weekly treatment. As the issue was explored, Hillary was able to acknowledge some secret pleasure in keeping her male therapist waiting for her. Further discussion revealed that this was an attempt at revenge, inasmuch as her father used to keep Hillary waiting for hours and always offered evasive answers when he was asked about it.

Later in treatment Hillary was able to realize that her heart problems were precipitated by having to wait long periods for her superiors to make decisions which affected her own schedule.

Reluctance to Pay Fees

Usually, though not always, a reluctance to pay fees expresses some resentment about the therapy and the therapist. Since fees are one of the few things that therapists can demand of patients, they may try to hurt the therapist by withholding what is wanted. Many, if not most, patients wish to be indulged like children and the idea of paying a fee to a parental figure seems ridiculous.

Ian, age 42, came to therapy on the recommendation of a friend. Ian was a classic cardiac personality. He needed to control everybody around him, was always trying to cope with intense hostile fantasies, had few intimate relationships but could not acknowledge his own dependency yearnings, and had several somatic problems including frequent breathlessness, high blood pressure, and chronic tiredness.

When Ian failed to pay his monthly fee for two months in a row, his therapist asked him about the difficulty. Ian bellowed, "You are supposed to take care of me. I'm not supposed to take care of you." His strong resistance to seeing the therapist as having needs of her own was present for some time. He wanted the therapist to be "an ideal mother" who would take care of him continually, the way his "own mother did not."

Silence

Silence in therapy, as in life situations, can have many meanings. It can be an expression of love such as is experienced by lovers after sex. It can also be an accompaniment of symbiotic merger, or can express defiance. As with any resistance, silence can be overdetermined.

> Although Jeanne, age 42, had angina, her reason for seeking therapy was because she had a strong aversion to sex. She could become very sullen, break out in hives, and often vomited when her husband wished to have sex with her. This had been going on during most of her 7-year marriage, and she finally developed enough courage to seek therapy.
>
> In her therapy with a male, she was silent, often for complete sessions. When the therapist did not force her to talk, she was eventually able to relax. After about 6 months of almost complete silence in treatment, Jeanne was able to find many reasons to account for her silences. Talking was like "putting out sexually" and she deeply resented it. It reminded her of working hard for her parents and not being appreciated. Jeanne had strong fantasies "to do just nothing" and being silent in therapy was her way to gratify this wish.

Overemphasis on the Present

It is difficult for most individuals to take responsibility for their problems. They would rather ascribe their difficulties to other individuals, to chance, or to some situational variable of which they have no control.

Cardiac personalities, who hate to acknowledge their own vulnerabilities, are quite adept at running away from themselves and instead spend much time fretting about an uncontrollable problem in their current reality.

> Ken, age 55, was referred to therapy by his physician. Ken had high blood pressure, suffered from insomnia and continual anxiety, and he was sexually impotent.

> In his treatment sessions, Ken spent most of his time talking about his lack of money. He had displaced his feelings of sexual inadequacy and his low self-esteem onto his financial problems. It took his therapist many months of weekly treatment before he could help Ken accept the idea that Ken should take a look at his own sexual anxiety, particularly as it was expressed in his relationship with his wife. Of more importance, Ken needed a great deal of help before he could talk about his childhood, which was very traumatic and at the root of his current problems. Like many individuals with painful pasts, Ken wanted to deny the importance of his early years.

Overemphasis on the Past

When current issues such as a heart condition and/or other personal and interpersonal problems are too painful to cope with, the patient can resist facing current issues by becoming obsessively preoccupied with the past.

> Louise, age 46, had many physical, emotional, and interpersonal problems. Her marriage was falling apart, her youngsters were difficult for her to manage, she was obese, and she had some cardiac symptoms. In her therapy the spent almost all of her time dwelling on her past, saying next to nothing about her marriage and family life and nothing about her physical problems. It took her therapist many months before she could help Louise face the dangers of talking about the present.

There are many forms of resistance other than the ones we have reviewed. Whatever form resistance takes, it is important for practitioners to keep in mind that resistances are present from the first phone call to the last session. All patients, no matter how much they want their lives to be different, fear change. All patients want to avoid the dangers and anxieties that self-exposure entails. This is particularly true for cardiac personalities who find exploring their emotions and conflicts very threatening. For therapy to be successful, cardiac personalities, like all patients, must be helped to accept resistances as a fact of therapeutic life, just as the use of defenses is a fact of daily living.

The Ubiquity of Countertransference

One of the impressive developments taking place in psychotherapeutic practice during the last two decades or so is a changed attitude toward countertransference. Until the mid-1970s countertransference tended to suggest those attitudes and activities of the therapist which interfered with the therapist's ability to understand and help patients. Current usage often includes all of the therapist's emotional reactions which are at work (Abend 1989). Slakter (1987) in his book *Countertransference* refers to countertransference as "all those reactions of the (therapist) to the patient that may help or hinder treatment" (p. 3).

Most contemporary therapists have moved away from the view of the therapist as a wise and mature healer ministering to a naive and disturbed patient. Now the perspective is of two equals who have similar vulnerabilities and conflicts working together to help resolve the patient's difficulties. Therapists of the 1990s seem to endorse Harry Stack Sullivan's (1953) idea that we are all "more human than otherwise."

Although countertransference reactions are ubiquitous, they, nonetheless, have to be understood by the therapist and their impact on the patient appreciated. In working with cardiac patients whose lives are "on the line," strong counter-transference reactions are inevitable. Many therapists want to quickly rescue their patients from harm and these therapists can become overactive with their advice. Others may become so frightened as they contemplate the patient's intensification of heart disease that they can withdraw. If these countertrans-ference reactions are not understood, they can harm the therapeutic process.

Examples of Countertransference

Positive countertransference

Psychotherapy usually proceeds well when the therapist likes the patient. Although positive countertransference is a desirable attitude, like a positive transference, it should be studied carefully (Fine 1982).

> Marvin was a married man in his early forties who spent a lot of his therapy discussing his arguments with his wife. Marvin felt that the "stress' he was under, and which contributed to his heart condition, came from his wife who was "controlling," "demeaning," and "critical."

> Marvin's female therapist felt a great deal of sympathy for him. Slowly she began to be quite critical of Marvin's wife. As she did so, Marvin felt very "supported." However, his arguments with his wife intensified, and eventually he and his wife separated. Marvin told his therapist, "I felt that you were my ally in the war and every time I was in a fight with my wife, you were the gun I needed."

> Marvin never did get to learn much about his unresolved problems with women. What he did get from therapy was "a gun."

Negative countertransference

Therapists usually have difficulty acknowledging their hostility toward their patients. Most feel obliged to love them constantly. Yet, therapists are human beings and can become frustrated by the patient's lack of progress, provoked by their criticisms, or bored by their complaints.

Acknowledging one's hostility toward the patient can often help the therapist understand how and why the patient is in interpersonal difficulty.

> Nora, age 41, was in treatment because it was determined by her physician and herself that her loneliness was part and

parcel of her heart condition. In her treatment with a male therapist, Nora would initially accept with enthusiasm her therapist's statements. However, within two sessions she would become critical of these statements and reject them. As the therapist found himself irritated with Nora's rejecting attitude and studied his reaction carefully, he was able to see what Nora did in her relationships with men. She would accept the men initially and then soon become critical and reject them. That was why she was so lonely.

Although it took some time to implement, the therapist was able to use his understanding of his countertransference reactions to help Nora.

One of the most common manifestations of repressed hostility in the therapist is the use of clinical diagnosis. It is what Erik Erikson (1950) refers to as *diagnostic name-calling*.

Oscar, a 58-year-old man, was in therapy for depression, work dissatisfaction, and unsuccessful relationships with women. After finding his first consultation with his female therapist encouraging, he changed his mind about her in the second interview and criticized her office, her demeanor, and her appearance. As his criticisms mounted, the therapist found herself referring to Oscar as "a pathological narcissistic character." Later when Oscar became still more critical, the therapist concluded that he was "a borderline personality."

Oscar eventually quit treatment. He could correctly say to the therapist, "I always felt you didn't like me." Because the therapist couldn't cope with her own hostility, she could not help Oscar cope with his.

When therapists cannot face something in themselves, they usually cannot help their patients face the same issue. Consequently, the better that countertransference reactions are understood by therapists, the better therapists can help their patients.

Common Mistakes of Therapists Treating Cardiac Personalities

Overzealousness and overactivity

As we have already suggested in our discussion of positive countertransference, therapists may want to rescue cardiac personalities. In their desire for a quick solution to their patients' difficulties, therapists can push them into activity, force them to confront issues prematurely, and ignore their resistances.

Although most therapists would not disagree with the notion that the best way to help patients is by providing a safe atmosphere in which they can freely talk, many therapists do not practice what they preach. In their eagerness to convince their patients that they are in competent hands, many therapists bombard the patient with "brilliant" interpretations and other interventions. Most patients feel overwhelmed with this and are rarely impressed.

Praise and Criticism

When therapists hear about the traumas and other misfortunes that their patients have experienced, it is tempting to express sorrow for their pains and aches and offer praise for their endurance. It is also tempting to criticize those patients who demean others but are self-righteous about their own behavior.

One of the difficult tasks in therapeutic work with cardiac personalities is suspending judgment and assessing the patient objectively. To see how the patient writes his or her own psychological script is not easy. To help the patient see this is even more difficult. However, praise and criticism turn patients into psychological children and they either feel forced to comply or compelled to rebel. They usually don't get much better with praise or criticism.

Making Rules and Offering Advice

It takes some time for the therapist to accept the fact that quiet, attentive, unobtrusive listening is what truly helps patients feel and function better. Many therapists, in their eagerness to help, give patients rules for living and advice on how to implement these rules. The patient's autonomy then goes underground, he or she feels belittled, and no real insight follows. Patients get better when they discover themselves, not when they are told how to live.

Making Promises

It is often tempting to reassure a cardiac personality who is suffering from many physical and psychological aches and pains. What experienced therapists have learned is that reassurance is rarely reassuring. Patients become suspicious of it when they don't have the data in front of them that makes recovery a sure thing. Secondly, patients know that when they give time and money to the tedious process of psychotherapy, much more is warranted than mere promises.

In the next several chapters we will consider in sharper detail some of the major themes in the cardiac personalities' dynamics and discuss some of the fine points that are helpful in treatment.

4

From
Omnipotence
to Competence

It will be recalled that one of the major characteristics of cardiac personalities is their intense desire to feel and be omnipotent. Unable to feel competent except for brief periods, constantly trying to ward off deep feelings of helplessness and vulnerability, not able to trust others fully and always fearful of rejection, cardiac personalities try desperately to control their universe by aspiring to the roles of kings and queens. Inasmuch as their omnipotent wishes are frustrated by reality constraints almost all of the time, cardiac personalities are usually unhappy people who find it quite difficult to adapt to the real world.

In this chapter we will discuss how the defense of omnipotence is expressed in the cardiac personality's love life, work relationships, and day-to-day interactions. We will also review some of the typical childhood experiences of the cardiac personality so that we can better appreciate how and why attempts to become omnipotent are an inevitable outcome in adult life. Vignettes portraying how omnipotence is expressed in transference reactions and resistive responses will be presented. We will also utilize case illustrations in order to demonstrate how the patient's grandiose behavior influences the therapist's countertransference reactions and is always a component of therapeutic technique. Manifestations of the patient's omnipotence will be presented as it emerges at different phases of treatment, and how the therapist attempts to help the patient reduce it will be discussed.

Omnipotence: A Disturber of Love Life

When grandiose individuals try to gratify omnipotent fantasies, they become very difficult spouses and lovers, and usually induce much unhappiness and irritation in their partners. Their pathological narcissism (Kernberg 1988, 1995) constantly antagonizes their partners who resent their egotism and lack of empathy. When their partners react with anger, cardiac personalities feel very hurt and weak, and to cope with their bruised feelings, become even more controlling. This, in turn, alienates the spouse further.

> Zachary, age 46, had two heart attacks, the importance of which he tried to belittle. When his wife, Adele, expressed her concern that Zachary was not taking sufficient care of himself, he became infuriated and told Adele to mind her own business. Adele felt very misunderstood and tried to show Zachary that her intentions were very honorable and loving. Projecting his own narcissism onto his wife, Zachary lectured Adele, frequently telling her, "You always want to be the boss. Why don't you want to cooperate with me?"

The more Adele showed concern about Zachary's condition, the more controlling Zachary became. The more controlling he was, the more his wife harangued him. The couple became involved in intense power struggles and needed marital counseling to try to maintain their marriage.

What frequently gets cardiac personalities into immense difficulty in their marriages is their infantile demandingness. Like many individuals who tend to ascribe parental qualities to their spouse, cardiac personalities have a strong propensity to assume that their spouse can and should be a 24-hour-a-day breast. When the marital partner cannot meet this inordinate demand, cardiac personalities are capable of temper tantrums, sulkiness, and rebelliousness.

> Yetta, a 54-year-old woman, had two bypasses by the time she was 45. A tense, driven woman, she made many demands on her husband, Boris. She wanted him to be more active in their sex life, take more initiative with domestic chores, and be more responsible with the children. She was very dissatisfied with Boris' income and frequently suggested ways he could better it.
>
> Although Boris tried valiantly to comply with Yetta's demands, he often found himself feeling resentful toward her. Therefore, he was often forgetful about chores and passive-aggressive in many areas of living. Yetta would then feel very hurt and not talk to Boris for hours at a time because she felt rejected and taken for granted. Boris would become outraged at this behavior and his passive-aggressive behavior increased.

Cardiac personalities frequently have difficulties in their sex lives. Feeling unsure about themselves as competent sexual partners, anxious about their sexual performance, and worried about gratifying their partners, cardiac personalities have two major ways to cope with their feelings of vulnerability and inadequacy: overactivity and underactivity (Offit 1995). In the first category are those individuals who become sexual addicts, constantly requiring sexual contact to bolster their low self-esteem. Frequently, they have extramarital affairs—not so much to give and receive love, but to reassure themselves that they are sexually competent human beings, something they constantly doubt. In the second category are those men and women who try their best to abstain from sex, often apprehensive that they will perform poorly and become undesirable partners. Occasionally, we see both coping mechanisms in one person.

> Wolf, a man of 52 years, was referred for psychotherapy by his cardiologist after Wolf informed the doctor that his wife was "very unresponsive" sexually and that her lack of responsiveness was causing him "enormous stress." As Wolf's problems unfolded in psychotherapy, he told his therapist that he "needed" to have sexual relations with his wife "at least once a day." If his wife, Carol, did not respond to his demands, he cursed her and occasionally attacked her physically. Often, he left home for days at a time to have affairs with other women.

> When Wolf returned home, he was very apologetic, contrite, and very self-effacing. During these periods he was not interested in having sex with Carol but instead wanted to be "a good boy."

One of the ways that researchers (Fine 1982, Strean 1985) who have investigated marital conflict have been able to pinpoint the major struggles of marital partners is to study their marital complaints. What has emerged is a virtual axiom, namely, the chronic marital complaint is an unconscious wish that protects the complainer. For example, the husband who avers that his wife is cold and frigid secretly wants such a wife; a warm and responsive woman would threaten him too much. Similarly, the wife who castigates her husband for being weak and passive secretly wants such a husband; a strong and active man would create too much anxiety for her.

What do cardiac personalities complain about when they discuss their spouses or criticize them directly? Almost anything! They are very quick to find fault with everything from domestic chores to sex and from money to gardening. This, of course, makes considerable sense when we recall that cardiac personalities are in constant pain (J. Novick and K. Novick 1991). To try to cope with their underlying depression and desperation, they attack the spouse (and/or others) and attempt to inflict the pain on the marital partner that they themselves feel.

> Veronica, a 48-year-old married woman, started psychother-
> apy after having experienced a major heart attack. In her
> therapy she spent almost all of the time demeaning her
> husband, David. She described David as "a wimp" who did
> not know "which end is up." She had criticisms of him as a
> wage earner, sexual partner, father, and conversationalist.
> When her therapist asked Veronica what she thought kept
> her in her marriage, Veronica matter-of-factly stated, "He's
> a good man. I love him. Just because he doesn't know how
> to be a husband is no reason to leave him!"

Experts on marital interaction (for example Kernberg 1995, Lutz 1964) have observed repeatedly the complementarity or fit of the two members of the dyad. Some examples of this fit are the complementarity of the sadist and the masochist, the dependent alcoholic and the nurturing spouse, and the deceiver married to the naive individual who enjoys, albeit unconsciously, being deceived (Waelder 1941). Emotional pathology is frequently a binding factor in a marriage if it provides for complementarity in the marital interaction.

Cardiac personalities usually "find" spouses who aid and abet their omnipotent fantasies. Often the spouse has unconscious omnipotent fantasies which are vicariously lived through the cardiac personality.

> Ulysses, age 51, was a corporation executive. He was referred for psychotherapy by his physician, who felt that his hypertension was related to his "intensely driven" behavior.

> In his therapy he told his therapist that he had a compulsion to achieve and could not stop himself, no matter how hard he tried. Overambitiousness was also apparent in almost every phase of living—with friends, in his recreational interests, and with his children. "I want to be the first and the best at everything," Ulysses frequently commented.

> As he reviewed his marriage, Ulysses gave his therapist many examples of how his wife, Ethel, encouraged him to work hard. Every time a well-paying job was mentioned in social conversation, Ethel would say, "Maybe you'd like that, honey?" If anyone accomplished anything in sports, Ethel commented, "You can do that, honey. Go to it!" In many ways Ulysses was a workaholic and Ethel was his main supporter in this venture.

Omnipotence at Work

A visit to almost any cardiac rehabilitation program will be an opportunity to meet with highly successful professionals, business executives, reputable academicians, and other accomplished men and women. It is rare to find an under-achiever in any of these programs.

Many men and women in our society measure their self-esteem by how much money they make and the status they achieve on the job. This is, of course, true of cardiac personalities, and more so. No matter what they achieve, they are never satisfied. There is always the possibility of doing better and that is why many of them become workaholics. Most of the time, cardiac personalities ascribe their 14 hours of work each day to the nature of the job, and they are usually un-aware of the demands they place on themselves.

> Theresa, age 39, was a physician who came for psychother-apy because, according to her own diagnosis, she was "suffering from symptoms of overwork." Theresa was constantly feeling tired, depressed, breathless, and had migraine headaches. As she described her work at a general hospital, it became quite clear that she was really making a lot of work for herself. She had enormous resistance to delegating responsibility to other professionals, got overinvolved in many areas of her patients' lives that were beyond her scope as an internist, and had to read and reread every medical journal she came across. When her therapist asked Theresa why she thought she was so overworked, she responded, "It's the nature of my job. I'm just a victim of circumstances." It took her many months of therapy before she could say, "I guess I feel like I'm a nobody unless I'm busy working."

Many cardiac personalities feel that they have no identity to speak of unless they are busy at work. Because they are full of self-doubts, they become compulsive perfectionists (Blatt 1995), as was observed in the case of Theresa. In addition, because cardiac personalities experience feelings of impotence unless they are in an omnipotent position, they are fiercely competitive. Anybody else's achievement is their failure. They and someone else cannot be successful at the same time. There is always a winner and a loser.

> Sam, a 65-year-old attorney, was describing to his therapist some of his feelings after he had just completed a successful closing on a house. "It was peaceful and pleasant and everybody was friendly. I would say that everybody, including the lawyers, were satisfied. I should have been happy, but I wasn't. Something was missing. I realized I missed a good fight. Even if I lose the fight, it's okay. Without a fight, I don't feel alive."

Although not a universal characteristic of cardiac personalities, what is often found among them at work is indecisiveness. Not confident of their own strengths, anxious that they might antagonize others, fearful of their own aggression, cardiac personalities can get into difficulty on the job because they do not trust themselves. Often they feel there is "a perfect decision," "an absolutely correct way" which they cannot seem to find.

> Rhoda was a 54-year-old executive director of a social agency. Although competent in many ways, she was always in a state of doubt about her abilities and decisions. Because of her lack of confidence in herself, she would ask staff and board members what they thought about various initiatives

she would take. Inasmuch as there was always disagreement among her colleagues, Rhoda could never come to a decision with ease. Work piled up, the agency began to decline in efficiency, and Rhoda was about to lose her job when she sought psychotherapy.

Just as arrogant and egotistic attitudes in marriage antagonize the spouse, the same attitudes provoke colleagues. Very often, when the cardiac personality is in a position of leadership, he has a tendency to act in an authoritarian manner. Feeling the necessity of controlling others lest they take a precarious sense of power away, the cardiac personality often gives orders in an undignified way to people.

> Quincy, a 50-year-old dean in a large metropolitan university, came for psychotherapy because he was constantly clashing with his colleagues. The arguments were stressful for him and he began to have cardiovascular symptoms. In his early interviews with his therapist, he said, "I know it's not the right way to be. But, I have to know everything, be on top of everybody, and not let anybody control me. If I feel that is happening, my knees wobble, I become tongue-tied, and I really fear I am going to be wiped out. Unless I'm the boss, I feel like I'm nobody."

Although cardiac personalities are always harboring a great deal of rage, they are often afraid of it. Consequently, they might inhibit themselves when normal assertiveness is required because they are not sure what kind of aggression might emerge. Fearful of speaking up, sometimes the cardiac personality fails to impress others and can lose a job.

> Peter, age 45, was referred to therapy by his physician after he lost his job and was showing high blood pressure and

other cardiovascular symptoms. In the therapy, he mentioned that he was in "a constant rage," so he "always shut up." Peter, though feeling very competitive and scornful of his colleagues, was afraid "they'd get to know" him. Therefore, he was inordinately quiet and was eventually labelled as an "odd ball" who had nothing in common with his colleagues. It took him many months of therapy to be more accepting of his aggressive fantasies and to talk about them rather than repress them.

As mentioned in Chapter 3, the cardiac personality usually has a punitive superego. Unable to enjoy her instinctual life because of an intense fear of regressing to an infant, the cardiac personality often works overtime to avoid the anxiety that normal pleasure and relaxation induces. Although the cardiac personality resents overworking, continuing the grind is rarely questioned.

Olive, a 44-year-old attorney, worked 16-hour days. Often she worked through the night. When she developed physical symptoms and her physician could find no organic basis for them, Olive was referred for psychotherapy. In her therapy Olive pointed out constantly that if she didn't work hard, she felt much guilt and shame. While this was being explored further, Olive commented, "If I don't work and just take it easy, I feel like an evil person who is getting away with murder." Olive learned much later in her therapy that she harbored many murderous fantasies. She really wanted to murder her punitive and demanding parents every time she "took it easy." Consequently she avoided pleasure and relaxation.

Omnipotence in Daily Life

When a piece of behavior bolsters self-esteem, the behavior emerges everywhere. Cardiac personalities, as we have reiterated, need to feel like supermen and superwomen in almost all areas of living lest they become, in their minds, weak insignificant children as they really did feel in their formative years.

Cardiac personalities have to be first everywhere. They seek heaps of attention and admiration in most of their interpersonal relations. They must tell the best jokes, the most dramatic stories, and they exhibit their achievements at every opportunity. When they do not receive the response they want, they can become very depressed.

> Nathan, a man of 57 years, came for therapy because he was deeply depressed and had many psychosomatic symptoms. Early in his therapy he told his therapist that he had no friends and felt very socially isolated. Although he presented himself to the therapist as a kind and considerate man, it was quite clear that not only did he dominate all conversations in which he was involved, but in addition he was very critical of his friends and always knew more than they did. Nathan's depression was a response to real rejection. He had to learn in his therapy how his provocative behavior alienated him from his peers.

The intense desire to conquer the world gets the cardiac personality into all kinds of difficulties. Eager to be Number One, he or she can fight the dictates of a strong superego and break the law.

> Mary, age 47, was seen in a mental health clinic connected with a court system. She had amassed a collection of speed-

ing tickets and as part of her sentencing had to go into therapy. She told her therapist, "I always have to speed. Sometimes I'm not really in a hurry but I have to beat everybody else on the road. If I don't, I feel I'm an insignificant person. It may not be logical, but that's the way I feel."

Cardiac personalities are often very intelligent people. With their rational minds, they know their omnipotent behavior and narcissistic wishes are inappropriate, but they frequently cannot monitor them without feeling wiped out.

Larry, a 40-year-old man who had two heart attacks, sought therapy because he had many phobias. One revealed his intense grandiosity. This was his phobia of movie theaters—he had to stay away from them. As this phobia was examined in his therapy, Larry confessed that unless he was guaranteed a good seat in advance, he could not and would not attend the movie. To sit in a seat that did not make him feel like a member of "the elite" was to force him "to feel like a bum." Rather than take that chance, he resisted going to the movies.

The difficulty that Larry experienced with the movies is similar to the problems that many cardiac personalities encounter in restaurants, in hospital emergency rooms, or whenever they have to join the crowd and be served on a "first come, first served" basis. If they do not get their food pronto, they are in a rage. If the doctor does not minister to them instantly, they are furious. And, if they are in a slow traffic lane, they will get out of it and get into a faster lane, even if doing so is illegal. Furthermore, when any of this behavior is questioned, they are indignant.

Karen, age 51, was in a group for cardiac patients. In session after session she told the group members how proud she was of "telling people off." She boasted about how she insulted waiters who did not serve her fast enough, cab drivers who did not drive to her liking, and others who did not gratify her narcissism. When one of the members of the group suggested that maybe her heart ailments had something to do with her constant desire to be treated like a member of royalty, she broke out into a temper tantrum and threatened to leave the group permanently.

Because the danger of losing the omnipotent position is considered so catastrophic by the cardiac personality, the individual can go to enormous extremes to salvage it. On a psychological level, losing the omnipotent position can be equivalent to death and/or becoming an orphan (Erikson 1950).

Jonathan, a man of 54 years, came to therapy because he was close to bankruptcy. The idea of not having much financial stability was making him feel very depressed which in turn caused him to drink excessively, and he had "unexplained" chest pain.

Living in a suburb of wealthy people, Jonathan "could not stand it" if one of his neighbors had a more expensive car, a nicer looking house, or a more lavish party. He spent a big part of every day finding ways and means to surpass his neighbors and even more time implementing his plans. Eventually, he was spending enormous time away from his business and large amounts of money in order to outdo his confreres. "To not be the most outstanding," stated Jonathan, "is to feel like an idiot."

When individuals doubt their strengths and have low self-esteem, they can become psychopathic in their behavior. The more they doubt their own potency, the more they have to exhibit themselves, and often in a questionable manner.

> Isadora, age 40, though a successful physician, always doubted her standing in professional and social communities. To bolster her self-image, she resorted to a lot of psychopathic behavior. She would arrange to have herself paged at concerts and other events so people would think she was a popular physician. At the country club, she would alter her scores in golf matches so that she could be the winner. In her church she would have higher donations announced than she actually gave.

> When Isadora's behavior was examined in therapy, she confessed, "I've always felt that I was a second class citizen, particularly next to men. If I was going to be a somebody and I really have wanted to be a somebody, I've had to be somebody else other than myself."

The Etiology of Omnipotence—Childhood Experiences

As we have stated several times, omnipotence should be regarded as a defense against pain. Feeling weak, helpless, and vulnerable, the individual protects himself or herself from feeling insignificant by behaving in a grandiose manner. Therefore, in examining the childhood histories of cardiac personalities, we should expect to see them laden with pain.

One of the most common childhood themes of cardiac personalities is that for a while the youngster felt quite loved and secure and then, rather abruptly, the secure status was taken away.

> Henry, age 60, whose heart condition developed shortly after a close friend of his committed suicide, told his therapist that the traumatic event reminded him of a childhood experience. He recalled that after greatly enjoying the first four years of his life, his brother was born. Henry felt very displaced by his brother. He believed that his brother was much more loved and admired and that he, Henry, "didn't have a chance" next to him. Whether he had crying jags, got depressed, or was provocative and aggressive, he was ignored by his parents and others. Feeling insignificant, Henry spent the rest of his life trying to be Number One in everything he undertook.

Rejection seems to be a frequent happenstance in the childhoods of cardiac personalities. What is important to keep in mind in assessing the histories of these patients is that their subjective reactions are the *sine qua non* in trying to understand their omnipotent defense. Sometimes they feel more rejected than they actually were. However, it is their own interpretation of life events which can help us better understand their grandiose orientation to living.

> Gloria, a young woman in her thirties, had a host of psychosomatic difficulties—migraine headaches, insomnia, gastrointestinal difficulties, and hypertension. As she reviewed her childhood history in her therapy, she talked extensively and with much affect about her brother who was severely handicapped and spent almost all of his life in a wheelchair. Gloria interpreted the excessive attention that her brother received as an indication of her worthlessness. Although her parents probably felt quite loving toward Gloria, she did not

experience them that way. Rather, she felt that "there was always something missing in me and I was never regarded too highly by my parents."

Another theme that frequently emerges in reviewing the childhood histories of cardiac personalities is that they were pressured to achieve. What often happened to them is if they did not excel in school, sports, or interpersonally, they were severely reprimanded. When children are the recipients of this kind of abuse, they question their own worth. To make sure they are valuable they can become compulsive achievers and workaholics.

> Frank, age 55, went into group therapy with heart patients after he suffered a heart attack. As the group were sharing their childhood histories with each other, Frank talked about his authoritarian father who berated him if he came only second or third in his class, scolded him if he hit a single in baseball rather than a home run, and demeaned him if he asked questions because he should have known the answers. As the group members listened to Frank, most of them recalled similar histories. One member concluded, "Parents should be told that the best way to help kids grow up and become a victim of heart disease is to push the hell out of them."

Though pressuring a child can be an important etiological variable in the formation of a cardiac personality, the opposite form of child rearing can also be a factor.

> Ethel, age 40, was in treatment for acute anxiety and many somatic complaints including some mild heart problems. In describing her childhood, Ethel commented, "My parents asked nothing from me. I felt that I never had to achieve

anything. After a while I felt I was an idiot and I had to prove otherwise by becoming a compulsive workhorse."

When children are reared in repressive atmospheres where sexual wishes and aggressive fantasies are not permitted, the children have to deny their essential humanness. When this occurs, self-hatred is inevitable because the child thinks human feelings are despicable. To compensate for feelings of ugliness and pervertedness, the child resorts to grandiose behavior.

> Donald, a man in his fifties, was in treatment for sexual impotence. He also had psychosomatic difficulties including a heart ailment. In describing his childhood, he recalled that both of his parents repudiated any sign of emotion; he lived "in an emotional refrigerator." Donald recalled that as a teenager he "hated living" and thought of suicide on many occasions. Later, to ward off inferiority feelings, he became "very pompous."

Omnipotence in the Therapeutic Setting

Those who have worked professionally with people in distress recognize that despite the suffering of these individuals, when they become patients in therapy, they always recapitulate their characteristic problems in their relationship with the therapist. Therefore, omnipotence is a constant theme in the transference reactions of cardiac personalities and in the ways they resist treatment.

Transference Reactions

At the beginning of psychotherapy, cardiac personalities, if they have resolved their resistance to becoming psychotherapy patients, tend to idealize the therapist and often feel they have met the perfect parent they have longed for all of their lives. Feeling protected and loved, they temporarily renounce some of their own "greatness," and project it onto the therapist. This "honeymoon phase" of treatment (Fine 1982) activates feelings of enthusiasm, optimism, and increased self-esteem in most patients.

Just as reality always frustrated the patient's quest for omnipotence, the reality of the therapeutic situation eventually necessitates the patient's recognizing that the therapist is not a perfect person. When this recognition occurs, the patient can become very critical of the therapist and feel the same disillusionment that he felt with his parents in early childhood.

It is important for the therapist not to be defensive when criticized by the patient. Otherwise, the therapist will be perceived as one who champions omnipotence and cannot accept imperfections as facts of life. If the therapist can permit herself to be criticized without countering or censuring, the cardiac personality can be helped enormously. Seeing that a professional can be vulnerable without being defensive or hostile, the patient may try to behave similarly.

> Constance, a woman in her mid-fifties, was in psychotherapy because of severe marital problems. Both in her marriage and in her relationships with colleagues at a hospital where she was a psychiatric nurse, Constance found herself in numerous power struggles. Easily hurt, Constance often went on the offensive and alienated many people.
>
> For the first 4 months of Constance's twice a week therapy, she was in an elated mood. She "truly loved" her female therapist, who seemed "loving, kind, bright, and empathetic." During this time Constance's relationship with her

husband improved a great deal and she did much better with her peers on the job.

During the fifth month of Constance's therapy, after her therapist announced that she would be going on a vacation, Constance's mood changed dramatically. She began to feel irritable everywhere and in addition demeaned her therapy and her therapist. She spent several weeks criticizing the therapist's grooming, office decor, manner of speech, "phony" attitude toward her patients, and she threatened to quit treatment on several occasions.

When Constance observed that her therapist did not and would not retaliate when attacked, Constance became less offensive. Slowly she began to compliment the therapist for "taking a lot of junk" and later stated, "I'm learning from you that making mistakes and having limitations is not a crime. It doesn't mean you are an idiot if you are imperfect."

When the patient can observe that the therapist is a member of the human race and therefore makes mistakes, has vulnerabilities, and does not know everything, the patient slowly identifies with this perspective. It is the first step in the move away from championing omnipotence as a way of life to accepting competence as a worthwhile *modus vivendi*.

One of the common transference reactions of cardiac personalities is to insist that the therapist has the capacity to be the type of parental figure who gratifies all of the patient's demands. Of course, if the therapist does attempt to indulge the patient, the latter believes omnipotence is an achievable way of life and continues to try to get more demands gratified. However, the responsible clinician, to help the patient mature and become weaned, attempts slowly to frustrate the patient's inappropriate demands.

> Barry, age 42, was a single man who sought therapy because he could never sustain a relationship with a woman. He was lonely and depressed much of the time and had several somatic symptoms.
>
> After about one year of therapy in which he made significant progress, Barry began to want a symbiosis with his female therapist. He felt that it was crucial to his therapy to call his therapist in between sessions in order "to chat," extend the therapeutic session beyond its usual 45 minutes, and to have detailed information on the therapist's personal life.
>
> When Barry's therapist did not gratify his requests, but subjected them to examination, trying to help him explore his motives for demanding what he did, Barry became enraged. He began to be very critical of the therapist and castigated her incessantly.
>
> It took Barry many months of twice a week therapy before he could learn to accept limited gratification in therapy without having temper tantrums. However, when he was better able to do so, for the first time in his life he could begin to form a close relationship with a woman and his somatic symptoms diminished in severity.

One of the most difficult times in the therapy of the cardiac personality for both patient and therapist is when the patient relives his very conflicted childhood in the transference and experiences the therapist as a sadistic, insensitive parent. The reason this stage of therapy is so oppressive for patients is that they really are inclined to believe that they are hated by a therapist who is out to get them. For therapists, it can be a painful time because they are ascribed qualities that are difficult for them to accept—sadistic, narcissistic, insensitive, uncaring, and so forth. Yet, it is a necessary stage of treatment for the cardiac personality—a time to "deposit toxic wastes" (Klein 1932).

> Anne, a 48-year-old woman, was in treatment because of a very conflicted marriage, intense difficulties with her teenaged children, vocational problems, and somatic difficulties.
>
> After trying unsuccessfully to seduce her therapist to indulge her in many ways—answer personal questions, gab on the phone between sessions, turn the therapy sessions into friendly tête-à-têtes, have an affair, and more, she regressed considerably. Anne quit working and stayed home in bed, sleeping. She withdrew from her husband and children and felt strongly that the therapy was a complete waste of time. The therapist, although initially alarmed by Anne's very infantile behavior, eventually realized that he had to live through Anne's misery with her without trying to analyze it away. When Anne realized that the therapist gave her the right to relive in the transference her chaotic past, she became much less belligerent and more cooperative.

Cardiac personalities, because they are very narcissistic, try to maintain a sense of omnipotence and omniscience in the treatment sessions. Very often they attempt to weaken the therapist's authority and expertise and turn the therapist into a patient. Then they project parts of themselves onto the therapist and try to make them appear weak and helpless.

It is very important for therapists who want to help cardiac personalities sustain their therapeutic relationships not to become defensive or offensive when attacked by the patient. Rather, they should attempt to "use the patient as consultant" (Strean 1970).

> Ben, age 52, was seen for a consultation by his wife's therapist. Because Ben was reluctant to have therapy for himself, he was invited to have a consultation in order to "help (his wife's) therapy be more meaningful to her."
>
> Like many narcissistic individuals, Ben used his interviews with the therapist to exhibit his intellectual prowess and sexual appeal (Kernberg 1995). When the therapist, a woman, responded neutrally to Ben's bragging and arrogance, Ben began to become very critical of her. He told her that he thought she needed therapy and that he could help her more than she could help him. When the therapist asked Ben what problems of hers he thought they should discuss, Ben became very anxious. Stammering and stuttering, Ben barely could say, "Why, why, your, your insecurity." Hearing this, the therapist asked further, "Could you tell me what parts of my insecurity you are referring to?" Again, Ben was startled but tried valiantly to enact the role of therapist and turn the therapist into a patient.
>
> The more the therapist could feel free to abdicate her own role of "knowing doctor" and behave like an equal to Ben, the less threatened Ben felt. After about ten interviews Ben could say, "You know, I'm learning that not being a know-it-all is a good way to behave. What I've learned from you, I'm applying to my own life and it works. I don't have to be a big shot all the time."

Treatment Resistances

As can already be inferred, cardiac personalities present many resistances in treatment, particularly when their own omnipotence is threatened. Inasmuch as being a patient in psychotherapy almost always punctures cardiac personalities' narcissistic and grandiose defenses, their resistances are formidable and frequent.

One of the ways that cardiac patients challenge the therapy and the therapist and thereby protect themselves is by defying the "ground rules of treatment." Patients may absent themselves from treatment, come late for interviews, or have trouble paying their fees. Sometimes a patient can refuse to cooperate with several of the therapist's requests simultaneously.

> Charlotte, age 51, was referred for psychotherapy by her physician after it was clear that she was quite depressed, resented her divorced status, had difficulty relating to her married daughter and son-in-law, disliked her job as a guidance counselor, and had numerous somatic complaints.
>
> After enjoying a "honeymoon" with her male therapist, which helped diminish her depression considerably, Charlotte was able to enjoy her job and her relationships much more. However, during the seventh month of her treatment, when her therapist expressed pleasure about Charlotte's therapeutic progress, Charlotte's elated attitude changed dramatically. Instead, she came to interviews in a very sullen mood, was late for most of them, "forgot" to bring her check to pay her monthly fee, and found excuses to miss several appointments.
>
> When the therapist confronted Charlotte about her lateness, absences, and delinquent payments, Charlotte became indignant. She told the therapist that he was "very authoritarian," "arbitrary" and "very critical." When the therapist did not challenge Charlotte's contemptuous attitude, Charlotte

began to feel guilty and depressed. Slowly the therapist was able to show her the similarity between her depression in the treatment situation and her depression in her day-to-day life. Charlotte could appreciate more than ever before how her depressed attitude masked many hostile fantasies and feelings.

As the therapist helped Charlotte verbalize her hostile feelings and wishes in the sessions, she resumed cooperating with the ground rules of treatment. Eventually she could face the fact that she resented all authorities because they all reminded her of her "arbitrary parents." Facing her feelings of hurt and rejection that her parents induced in her, Charlotte needed her omnipotent defense much less.

As we have stressed, the cardiac personality tries to reinforce her omnipotence in the treatment situation because of the pain anticipated if she reveals her "true self" (Winnicott 1971). However, another way to protect her grandiose defense is by idealizing the therapist. The patient hopes that by praising the therapist and repeatedly noting his superb therapeutic talents, the therapist will not try to disrupt her tenuous psychological balance. In effect, the patient tries to gratify the therapist's omnipotent position so that she will be able to maintain her own omnipotent position.

Drew, a man in his early forties, was being seen in an outpatient clinic of a hospital following the examination by a physician who felt quite certain that Drew's high blood pressure and other cardiac problems were caused by stress.

Drew was very cooperative with the therapist, helping him better understand the stressful situations in which Drew was involved and how he experienced them. In fact, Drew did everything he could to be "a good patient" and continually praised his male therapist for being "sensitive," "empathetic," and "perceptive."

When it dawned on the therapist that he was being subtly manipulated, he decided to explore with Drew what his ingratiating attitude was all about. In his characteristic manner Drew "confessed" that it was "very important" that he and the therapist "get along with each other as well as possible."

It took several months of twice a week therapy for Drew to realize that he spent much time and energy in and out of therapy being very ingratiating. He eventually learned that his deferential attitude helped him "to be highly esteemed by others." If he did not have other people's high regard (and feel omnipotent), he was worried that he would become "a helpless idiot," which was the way he experienced himself throughout his childhood and adolescent years.

After Drew could better understand the function of his idealizing the therapist, he could face how weak and vulnerable he felt.

When cardiac personalities are helped in therapy to face how much pain and helplessness they have felt most of their lives, their omnipotent defense usually recedes and they become more interpersonally related. However, this is hardly ever a smooth process. In most psychotherapy, the patient takes one or two steps forward and then one or two backward (Fine 1982). This is particularly true for the cardiac personality, who very much needs to protect himself or herself from feeling vulnerable. Consequently, after he makes progress and seems more relaxed, he might follow this up by becoming intensely anxious and very resistive in his therapy.

> After Esther, age 60, had made much progress in her therapy
> by becoming aware that her supercilious attitude was a
> strong defense against strong feelings of inferiority, her
> demeanor in her therapy changed considerably. Instead of
> being relatively open with her feelings and warm toward her
> female therapist, Esther became quite removed. She intellec-
> tualized most of her productions and discussed essentially
> nonconflicted issues. When the therapist tried gently to
> remark about Esther's shift of attitude in the treatment,
> Esther dismissed her efforts. Being confronted with her
> resistance, Esther began to come late for some sessions and
> also missed a few.

> It took Esther many months before she could feel safe
> enough to share her feelings and conflicts again. She con-
> fided to her therapist that "trusting another person is a hard
> job."

Countertransference Issues with Omnipotent Patients

One of the reasons that cardiac personalities have not been
clearly understood nor fully appreciated as patients who can
be helped in psychotherapy is because they can arouse strong
countertransference reactions in clinicians. Further, as we
mentioned in Chapter 3, it is only within the past decade or so
that countertransference has been viewed as a constant
variable in the treatment, having as much influence as transference and resistance do on therapeutic outcomes (Abend 1989,
Strean 1993a).

Inasmuch as many clinicians have many omnipotent

fantasies of their own, it is often difficult for them to face patients who expose what they are trying to deny in themselves. One way that therapists cope with the anxiety aroused in themselves on seeing neurotic behaviors and attitudes in their patients which they, themselves, harbor, is by reassuring their patients that the material being discussed is mature and healthy. In this way therapists can deny their own problems and concomitantly deny the patient's.

> Each time Fred, a patient in his early fifties, mentioned in his therapy sessions that he was "hyper-ambitious and over-competitive," his therapist told him that his behavior was normal and that he was being too critical of himself. Although Fred's anxiety diminished for a short period, it would return and Fred would again talk about his unacceptable ambitiousness and competition. However, the therapist would again assure Fred that he was "normal."

> It was not until the therapy reached a stalemate and Fred was threatening to leave it that the therapist began to recognize his own countertransference problem. After discussing the case with a colleague, the therapist was able to recognize that by not permitting Fred to talk about his omnipotent fantasies, he was protecting himself and concomitantly stopping Fred from growing. With his new insight, the therapist began to listen rather than reassure. This helped Fred eventually face his own grandiosity and resolve most of it.

A countertransference reaction that is not discussed very much in the psychotherapeutic literature (nor in the medical literature) is the sexualized countertransference. In his recent book, *Love Relations: Normality and Pathology*, Otto Kernberg (1995) has averred:

> Although the countertransference as a factor in the
> formulation of transference interpretations has been
> receiving growing attention in the literature...far
> more has been written about aggressive counter-
> transference than about erotic countertransference.
> The traditionally phobic attitude toward the counter-
> transference, which has changed only in recent dec-
> ades, still operates with regard to the [therapist's]
> erotic response to the erotic transference. [p.116]

One of the major anxieties of therapists who fear acknowledging and examining their erotic countertransference
reactions is that they worry they will act out their own sexual
wishes. In my research on therapists who do have sex with
their patients (Strean 1994b), I learned that therapists who
have sex with their patients seldom worry about it in advance,
and clinicians who worry about acting out sexually seldom do.
Nonetheless, the fear of acting out sexually usually masks a
wish to do so. If therapists are courageous enough to acknowledge their own sexual wishes, they can be more helpful
to their patients.

> Grace was an attractive woman in her mid-thirties who was
> being seen by a young male therapist in a mental health
> center. Grace had a history of depression, pressure in her
> chest, and also experienced many unfulfilling love affairs in
> which she acted very masochistically and self-destructively.
> After several months of twice a week therapy, Grace's
> depression diminished, her relationships with men improved,
> and her feeling of self-confidence in her job as an editor
> increased.
>
> As Grace became more expansive in her day-to-day life, she
> also became more enthusiastic in her therapy and was

moderately seductive with her therapist. At first her therapist was oblivious to Grace's seductive overtures, not allowing himself to give any meaning to or experience any feeling about Grace's comments concerning the therapist's "lovely blue eyes," "melodic voice," "gorgeous clothes" and "sensitive disposition." However, when Grace told the therapist that she was "very much in love" with him and "would like to have sex" with him, he had to listen!

Although the therapist was aware of Grace's erotic transference, he handled his discomfort with it by making many genetic interpretations. He told Grace that she had a deep yearning for a giving father and that accounted for her "interest" in him. The therapist also informed Grace that her feelings toward him were "a resistance that was interfering with therapeutic progress."

Insensitive to Grace's deep yearning to be appreciated as an adult sexual woman, the therapist was surprised when Grace started to miss sessions and come late to most. He was shocked when Grace became very rageful toward him and told him he was "a pompous ass" who did "not know much about women or therapy."

Although the therapist finally did bring the case of Grace for consultation with a more experienced clinician, he was not able to allow himself to face his own uncomfortable feelings that were stimulated by his sexual interest in Grace. She left treatment prematurely.

The case of Grace and its outcome is a very instructive one. It helps us appreciate the fact that every human being wants to be accepted for herself as she is in the present. Grace needed to have an opportunity to express her fantasies about what she wanted to do with the therapist. This would have helped her get in touch with her yearnings, resentment, and many other feelings that were causing her depression and poor relationships with men. The therapist, frightened to hear about Grace's wishes, fears, hurts, and angers really rejected her by implying, "You don't love *me*! You love your father!" Grace felt rejected by this implication and therefore she rejected the therapist.

We also learn from the work with Grace that therapeutic technique is always based, at least partly, on the therapist's current countertransference position (Jacobs 1986, Renik 1993, Strean 1995b). Therapists can rationalize their use of therapeutic techniques with interesting concepts without taking into consideration how much their current counter-transference position is governing their interventions. This is why the conscientious therapist always tries to study his countertransference reactions and enactments.

As has already been implied, in dealing with the cardiac personality's omnipotence in the treatment situation, the therapist is frequently experienced as an enemy who is trying to take away the patient's power. To protect himself from being weakened, the patient often tries to weaken the thera-pist. Many therapists experience the patient's attempt to weaken them as a personal injury and become vindictive. A power struggle between patient and therapist ensues and it frequently does not get resolved.

> Harvey, age 57, was being seen by a female therapist because of several somatic difficulties, sexual problems, and conflicts with colleagues at his law firm. Although Harvey and his therapist worked well together for close to a year, when the therapist announced that she was going on a

vacation, the relationship between them changed dramatically. Harvey, to defend against his feelings of rejection and impotence, told the therapist that he decided that he would not return to therapy after her vacation because therapy had "reached a point of diminishing returns."

The therapist, taking Harvey's rejection personally and not understanding his motives, became very arbitrary and authoritarian and told Harvey that "it was necessary" for him to continue his treatment. Harvey, feeling weakened already, did not warm up to his therapist's mandates. Instead he did not show up for his last session before his therapist's vacation and did not resume his therapy.

The case of Harvey reminds us once again that the cardiac personality is constantly trying to maintain his grandiose position. When it is questioned, the patient feels powerless, helpless, and frequently angry. One of the ways the patient copes with the puncturing of his narcissism is to attack the therapist.

If the therapist does not take the slings and arrows of the patient's past too personally but tries to empathize with the patient, she becomes a very helpful role model. Seeing the therapist as a vulnerable human being with limitations of her own, the patient can slowly renounce his own omnipotence, explore his feelings of weakness, and uncover their roots. As the patient feels accepted by the therapist for who he really is, he begins to like himself more. Slowly he enjoys becoming a human being with ups and downs, with successes and failures in love, work, and everyday interactions. The tortured position of King becomes less appealing and competence is championed as omnipotence is relinquished. As the patient's stressful moments are lessened, his physical health usually improves.

5

From Rage
to Healthy
Assertion

In 1967, Peter Sifneos, a psychiatrist researching psychosomatic disease, coined a term to describe an individual's inability to experience or express emotions: *alexithymia* (literally "without words for emotions"). When alexithmic patients do mention experiencing an emotion and are questioned about it, they are generally not able to describe what they are feeling. Often they are merely aware of physical sensations.

Another psychiatrist, Henry Krystal (1979), in describing his therapeutic work with patients who suffer from alexithymia, pointed out that those patients who do not experience their emotions fail to attain a sense of aliveness. However, because they are constantly holding back affects, albeit unconsciously, the stress and strain mounts and they eventually become full of rage. Rage seems to be the only emotion they can consciously experience and either they are affectless or become explosive and rageful.

As we have noted in earlier chapters, one of the major characteristics of cardiac personalities is their inability to experience a full range of human emotions. However the vast majority of them harbor a great deal of hostility but have considerable difficulty knowing what to do with it. In many ways they can be said to be suffering from alexithymia.

What accounts for the intense rage in the cardiac personality? As we discussed in Chapter 4, when omnipotent wishes are powerful and pervasive, then the individual is going to feel constantly frustrated because reality rarely and consistently gratifies omnipotent wishes. Feeling deprived, the cardiac personality wants to attack those who do not gratify his or her grandiose wishes. When cardiac personalities do not feel omnipotent, they react with helplessness, vulnerability, and humiliation. Consequently they want to hurt those who have hurt them.

Usually when individuals have to cope with much rage toward the world, they have a great deal of unresolved hostility toward their parents that started in infancy or soon after. When cardiac personalities discuss their early histories, they often report that they are products of tense, anxious households where both father and mother had difficulty in relaxing, loving, and being empathetic (Levant 1995).

Bowlby (1969,1973,1980), in his three volume work on attachment and loss, shows that when a young child is not the recipient of consistent, tender, love and care, he or she goes through a series of predictable phases—protest, desperation, and detachment. In extreme cases, the child's body deteriorates and the youngster can die. In most cases, however, the child represses his despair, ceases crying, and withdraws from the world until he feels safe enough to protest again.

Cardiac personalities, because they have not enjoyed early

wholesome attachments, are constantly protesting against a world of people whom they experience as frustrating parents. They cannot allow themselves to feel their sadness and despair just as they could not in childhood. They become affectless until they explode in rage.

Rage for many cardiac personalities is what makes them feel alive and strong. They feel they are "a somebody" when they are raging at spouses, colleagues, friends, and strangers.

What seems so apparent about the childhoods of cardiac personalities is whenever they felt alarmed, afraid, frustrated, or anxious, their task was to repress and deny their feelings and come out angry and fighting. To acknowledge their feelings led to disapproval and withdrawal of love from parents (Levant 1995). Consequently, for cardiac personalities to experience feelings other than anger is to feel shame, which is very difficult, if not impossible, for them to tolerate. As Steven Krugman (1991) pointed out in a paper, "Male Vulnerability and the Transformation of Shame," shame is the emotional response to feeling exposed as inadequate, insufficient, dirty, vulnerable, and helpless. Indeed, shame is so excruciating to certain individuals, Krugman wrote, that it can drive them to instantaneous explosions of rage and violence—anything to escape unbearable feelings of vulnerability and humiliation.

Trying to Cope with Rage

As my colleagues and I have worked with cardiac personalities in therapy, we have observed that in addition to alexithymia, our patients both during their childhoods and also in later years, have tried to cope with their rage in a variety of ways. Some "turn the rage against the self" (A. Freud 1946) and become critical of themselves for a while. Because criticism from within or without is usually unbearable to the cardiac personality, the ensuing shame and humiliation can lead to feelings of depression.

In depression the patient feels sad, hopeless, helpless, and guilty. Invariably he or she feels a low sense of self-esteem. Margaret Mahler (1966) has described a developmental basis for this narcissistic vulnerability. She attributes it to the parents' (particularly the mother's) lack of acceptance and emotional understanding during the first two years of the child's life. This deprivation leads to the child's ambivalence toward the parents and finally to the affect of depression. As the child's self-esteem diminishes, he or she requires a great deal of outside reassurance to feel loved and acceptable. Mahler's thesis helps us understand better how cardiac personalities, with their fragile self-esteem, become depressed when they lose external support.

Jacobson (1971), who has also noted the intense aggression in depressed individuals, views their self-criticism as an expression of anger. This anger, she suggests, was part of the child's original attitude toward the parents when it was first experienced by the youngster, but it becomes directed inward.

As cardiac personalities review their early years with their therapists, many of them present vignettes where they wanted to be treated like naughty children. There seems to be within them an unconscious wish for punishment for their hostile wishes and deeds (Brenner 1959).

We have also observed a great deal of passive-aggressive behavior in cardiac personalities. Rather than directly expressing their aggression, which fills them with much ambivalence, cardiac personalities can get involved in being provocative under the guise of joking or debating. They can be forgetful, get into accidents, or make slips of the tongue, all of which can exasperate other people.

Having noted the difficulties that cardiac personalities have with their expression and tolerance of emotions—either they are in a rage or feel empty—explains, in many ways, why they have conflicts in so many of their interpersonal relationships. Either they are inclined to "tell people off" or often they feel nothing. They cannot feel free too often to assert themselves normally. As one cardiac patient of mine poignantly stated, "If I just talk, I fear I won't be heard. Either I have to make a big noise and become belligerent or I don't feel like saying anything."

Let us now take a look at some of the problems with rage which cardiac personalities experience in their marriages, work, and in other interpersonal situations.

Rageful Love Lives

Many, if not most, cardiac personalities fear emotional intimacy. Although the lack of intimacy in their lives makes them feel very lonely, despite their protests they would rather be angry. To be loving and close to a mate or partner often makes them feel like the helpless, vulnerable child of their pasts. To feel strong, to feel like a person, in their minds requires of them much belligerence and animosity.

As Kernberg (1995) has suggested, in order to enjoy a love relationship, both partners must be able to identify with each other and step into each other's shoes. In addition, he points out that a mature love relationship involves mutual tenderness. States Kernberg, "The feeling of tenderness is an expression of the capacity for concern about the love object. Tenderness expresses love for the other and is a sublimatory outcome of reaction formations against aggression" (p. 35).

May (1969) has discussed the importance of "care" as a prerequisite for mature love. Care, he has suggested, "is a state composed of the recognition of another, a fellow-human being like oneself, of identification of one's self with the pain or joy of the other; of guilt, pity, and the awareness that we all stand on the base of common humanity from which we all stem" (p. 289).

Balint (1948) described a true love relationship as including idealization, tenderness, and a special form of identification within which the "interests, wishes, feelings, sensitivity, shortcomings of the partner attain—or are supposed to attain—about the same importance as one's own" (p. 115).

The commitment, care, trust, tenderness, mutuality, and flexibility that are necessary for a satisfying love life are limited in cardiac personalities. To commit and care feels like one is being ignobly dominated. To trust in a tender way risks feeling exploited. To identify and temporarily merge with the other is to risk being decimated. When cardiac personalities begin to feel just a little care and trust, they have to destroy it by becoming angry.

> Irma, a woman in her early forties, was in marital counseling because of frequent altercations with her husband, Ben. In her initial consultation with her therapist, Irma lamented, "We fight about everything—money, sex, friends, politics, and in-laws. We even fight about when I should take my medicine for my heart problems."

> As Irma and her female therapist discussed the specifics of

her arguments with Ben, a constant theme emerged. Every time Irma and Ben "made up" after an argument, Irma would feel "soft, sexual, and warm." When Ben noticed this and expressed pleasure with Irma's loving demeanor, Irma became rageful. She would think of the many times Ben had appeared "too confident" of her love and "too cocky" about his attractiveness to her.

With further therapy, Irma was able to recognize that whenever she felt soft and loving, she felt like "a little girl who could be exploited by a tyrannical parent." The more she explored this idea, the more she realized that to prevent herself from feeling like a submissive and vulnerable child, she would unconsciously arrange to become "a dominant, angry bitch, stronger than any father or mother."

As Moses-Hrushovski (1994) has suggested, many individuals hide behind power struggles as a defense. Like Irma, if they are not involved in an angry power struggle, they feel a loss of identity and a sense of defeat. To feel potent, they must aggressively demean their mates. As previously suggested, normal assertiveness feels too weakening for them.

Many cardiac personalities use sex for conquest and domination. As Avodah Offit (1995) has stated in *The Sexual Self: How Character Shapes Sexual Experience*, "Parents have unabashedly expected them to achieve in sports, business, politics. [Therefore] they are molded to become competitors in every aspect of life, like thoroughbred horses" (p. 95).

Cardiac personalities, to feel secure and dominant, try to make their sexual partners into servants. Then, when the demeaned servant or slave seems unappealing and lacking in eroticism, this can justify the patient's wish to have an extramarital affair.

John, age 48, was referred for therapy by his physician because he could not decide whether to leave his wife, Betty, and move in with his paramour, or vice versa. His indecision was causing insomnia, heart palpitations, headaches, and other symptoms.

In his sessions with his male therapist, John spent much of his time contemptuously demeaning and deriding his wife for being unappealing sexually. When the therapist asked John what was unappealing about Betty, John was stumped. Although it took him several months to realize it, John was finally able to say, "I guess I make her into my fat mother, even though she isn't fat. Then I have to move away from her."

The dynamics observed in the case illustration of John, like virtually every phenomenon occurring in the lives of cardiac personalities, may be seen in women as well as men.

Karen, age 51, was being seen in a family agency so that she could resolve some marital problems. In most of her sessions with her female social worker, she used the time to complain about her husband, Dan. She spoke constantly of his inability to assert himself, his passivity, and his lack of sexual appeal.

Several months after she had been in treatment, she confessed that she was having an affair with a neighbor. She realized that she could not tell the social worker about the affair because she felt the worker would think negatively of her. After Karen realized that she was making the therapist a judge (in reality an embodiment of her own superego) and could take some responsibility for her projections, Karen began to face her marital conflicts more directly.

> Karen eventually observed that closeness and intimacy with Dan made her feel weak. By "knocking" him, and making him feel weak, she could feel much stronger. Realizing that her affair was motivated more out of a wish to feel strength, she began to move closer to Dan.

One of the major causes for rage in the marriages of cardiac personalities is they have a strong tendency to project parts of themselves which they do not like onto their marital partners and then attack the partners for these characteristics. As Kernberg (1995) has stated:

> Unacknowledged and intolerable aspects of the self are projected onto the partner to protect an idealized self-image. Unconscious provocation of the partner to comply with the projected aspects of the self is matched by attacks on and rejection of the partner thus misperceived. [p. 144]

Although projecting part of what is unacceptable and anxiety-provoking to the self is a universal characteristic of most marriages, and of many interpersonal relationships in general, cardiac personalities who find it extremely difficult to tolerate their own vulnerabilities and imperfections tend to use this defense more often than most individuals do.

Rage at Work

In his book *Troubled Men*, Reuben Fine (1988) points out that the present-day idea that work can make people happy is a novel one in human history. Aristotle did not think so, nor, for many centuries, did the Christians look upon work as anything but an interference with God. In fact, in Christian mythology, work is punishment for humanity's sins. Fine suggests that in current society, work for many individuals is more of a curse than a blessing.

Inasmuch as the workday occupies a large percentage of most people's waking hours, how an individual copes with the work situation will have an enormous impact on his or her physical and mental health. Cardiac personalities, with their workaholic orientation, their strong desire for recognition and admiration, their deep yearning for achievement and advancement, and their championing of perfection, are inevitably going to experience deep dissatisfactions in their work relationships. As we now realize, when cardiac personalities are dissatisfied, they either repress their feelings or have to cope with intense and pervasive anger.

In *Anger: The Struggle for Emotional Control in America's History*, Carol and Peter Stearns (1986) produce much evidence that "without question, anger remains in the workplace" (p. 143). They also suggest that because so many men and women have to inhibit their expressions of anger, mental and physical problems are frequent. A strong positive correlation continues to exist between work satisfaction and physical and mental health (Fine 1990). In one 15-year study of aging (Palmare 1969), the strongest predictor of longevity was work satisfaction. In Gardell and Johansson's (1981) *Working Life: A Social Science Contribution to Work Reform*, this point was reaffirmed:

> There is some convergence around the Freudian definition of well-being as the ability to work, love, and play, around the idea of freedom from distressing symptoms (gastric discomfort, inability to sleep,

etc.) around veridicality of perception, and around
positive affect towards self and toward life. [p.19]

Inasmuch as many individuals feel they must behave
masochistically toward superiors and colleagues at work,
undischarged anger is one of the major causes of heart disease
in the workplace (Williams 1993).

Lloyd, age 46, had suffered from two heart attacks. Although
he changed his lifestyle considerably after the second heart
attack, exercising daily and watching his diet carefully,
Lloyd continued to have angina and other cardiac symptoms.

Pleased that his cardiologist referred him for psychotherapy,
Lloyd spent most of his time in the therapy sessions with his
male therapist talking about his fears and anxieties at work.
An assistant director in a social agency, Lloyd felt continually harassed by the director, a man 10 years his senior. The
director, a demanding, sadistic man, used Lloyd as a scapegoat and continually yelled at him. Lloyd compliantly took
the boss's constant berating but suffered inwardly.

It was only after Lloyd could feel less afraid of his own rage
and more aware of how he was making the boss a big daddy
that his symptoms diminished. As he felt less like a mistreated little boy and more of a man with "a little boy boss"
did Lloyd's cardiac problems diminish.

Kernberg (1995), in a chapter on masochistic pathology in
his book *Love Relations*, states:

In my experience, women's masochistic love relations are more frequent than men's, but men's masochistic submissiveness in the workplace is proba-

bly more frequent than women's. I believe that male therapists in particular may underestimate the extent to which masochistic patterns in men's submissive behaviors are played out in the workplace. Again, objective discrimination against women in the workplace must be distinguished from men's widespread, culturally adaptive submissiveness to authority and power. [pp. 133-134]

Where masochistic submissiveness becomes almost a *modus vivendi* in the workplace may be observed in the way many African-American men and women feel compelled to cope with their superiors. As Chet Walker (1995), a former basketball great, describes in *Long Time Coming: A Black Athlete's Coming-of-Age in America*, many African-Americans have had to say, "Yes, sir" to a 6-year-old white boy. Walker talks about how this self-effacing masochistic attitude can do much damage to the self-image and turn a person into "a monster."

What is pertinent about the African-American's experience in the workplace is that the demeaned position "required" of them, and the consequent need to cope with much suppressed rage, may have some relationship to heart disease. According to the United States Department of Health and Human Services (1988), African-Americans have an almost one third greater chance of high blood pressure than whites. Furthermore, high blood pressure is generally more severe among African-Americans than whites as is heart disease in general.

Another dynamic in many work situations which is a factor in heart disease is competition. As we have noted, the cardiac personality strives to be Number One in anything he or she undertakes. Work is no exception.

Madeline, a woman in her late twenties, was referred to an outpatient psychiatric facility because of chronic headaches, insomnia, heart palpitations, and other somatic symptoms.

In her work as an elementary school teacher, she was well-liked by the children, her peers, and supervisors. However, Madeline never seemed satisfied with herself and constantly thought how she could do much better. This was not an idle thought. Madeline obsessed about her shortcomings and made herself miserable.

During her fourth month of treatment with a male therapist, Madeline had a dream in which she was yelling and screaming at several of her colleagues. Her associations to the dream revealed that she was in active competition with them and resented anything that any one of them achieved. It was not until Madeline could face that she was making her colleagues the siblings of her past whom, in many ways, she wanted out of the family that Madeline could relax a little on the job.

In *Hostility and the Heart*, Redford Williams (1993) gathered a great deal of epidemiologic research that clearly demonstrated that job strain can set the stage for heart disease to develop. Job strain, he pointed out, is a form of stress wherein the individual feels very angry about situations and people but this stress cannot be controlled. States Williams:

> A tension-filled workplace is a significant factor in cardiovascular disease. What really makes a job hard on the body as well as on the mind is the combination of high psychological demands, such as pressure to meet deadlines, and a low level of control over work circumstances—what researchers call "decision latitude." [p. 71]

Anger in Everyday Situations

The readiness of human beings to be hostile to each other is one of the greatest problems of mankind. Examples of hostility in everyday life are to be found everywhere—tyrannical rule still persists in many countries of the world; rates of violent crime, divorce, and child abuse keep soaring. However, the fact that brutality has been so prevalent throughout history and continues to be so does not mean that it is basic to human nature. Our observations of other species would not offer support for such a contention. As Leon Saul (1976), in *The Psychodynamics of Hostility*, has suggested:

> With the nearly singular exception of man, sadistic cruelty and murder within a species is all but unknown in the rest of the animal kingdom. You would have to descend to the harvester ant to see anything even remotely like it. A close look at man's behavior reveals that it has all the earmarks, not of nature, but of sickness, of psychopathology. [p. 6]

Very often we disregard the fact that ours is "a hate culture" (Fine 1982). People find it easier to compete than to cooperate, to condemn rather than to praise, to hate rather than to love. In many ways, cardiac personalities may be regarded as conforming members of our society because of their intense desire for power, victory, and achievement. Like many others, they feel that if they don't aggressively push others out of the way, they will be pushed.

> Nicholas, a man in his mid-sixties, arrived at one of his therapy sessions with a black eye and a broken nose. While

waiting in line to buy a ticket for the movies, the person behind him bumped into him. Nicholas yelled at the man and a fistfight ensued.

As Nicholas explored the why's and wherefore's of the incident with his therapist, he said angrily, "I can't stand it when anybody gets ahead of me. It makes me feel insignificant. I'll be damned if I'm going to let anybody make me feel insignificant. I'll make him insignificant first."

Nicholas, like many cardiac personalities, felt inferior to anybody he could not surpass and powerless next to anybody he could not overcome. Consequently, he was frequently in a rage because like all mortals he was often not Number One in many interpersonal situations.

An issue which often comes up in therapeutic work with cardiac personalities is that despite their inordinately strong drive to gain prestige, power, and perfectibility, the enormous strain which this induces creates a great deal of hostility in them. Because this hostility is not usually conscious, it affects the body. As will be recalled, as early as 1939, Franz Alexander demonstrated that individuals who force themselves to carry responsibilities while concomitantly harboring powerful longings to withdraw and flee from such burdens often develop high blood pressure.

Olga, a woman in her late thirties, was being seen in a family agency for marital and family difficulties. One day while hurrying to her appointment with her therapist, she found herself becoming breathless and thought she was going to faint.

In her session with the social worker, Olga described similar incidents and then pensively remarked, "If I keep going this way, I'm going to end up with a heart attack."

It took Olga many more months before she could realize that she was feeling enormous resentment because of her many responsibilities. She was a housewife, a mother of three, a full time secretary, and an active member of her community. Like many cardiac personalities, Olga was repressing her rage and continually striving to do many things at once perfectly.

Olga's situation helps us understand better why heart disease is the number one killer of women and that more than half of all Americans who die each year of cardiovascular problems are women (U.S. Department of Health and Human Services, May 1988).

Just as overburdened people like Olga like to believe they are victims of circumstance and that the burdens they experience are being imposed on them by others, the same dynamic occurs with individuals who find themselves continually faced with hostile encounters. These individuals contend that the rest of the world is hostile and that they have to protect themselves. What is often overlooked by these men and women, and sometimes by their therapists as well, is that individuals who are continually involved in hostile encounters are unconsciously attracted to them.

Peter, age 75, was a psychologist who had retired from practice as well as from the presidency of a major professional organization. In therapy because of his many somatic problems as well as suffering from a major depression, Peter told his therapist, "I don't miss my practice but I sure as hell miss the presidency. But you know what I miss about the presidency? I miss the fights. I realize how much fighting has thrilled me."

Fighting in our culture is often rewarded highly. Boxers and wrestlers get paid much more than social workers and teachers. The "hood," prototype of the American gangster, has become a symbol of male virility and machismo throughout the world. The most extreme examples of antisocial behavior—even perpetrators of violent crime—are often perceived as heroes (Offit 1995) and cardiac personalities constantly aspire to be viewed as heroes.

You've Got to be Taught to Hate

In the musical "South Pacific," a song with a moving melody tells us that, "You've got to be taught to hate." Although all human beings are endowed with both sexual and aggressive drives, to be hostile, hateful, or destructive is something we learn. Many people, particularly cardiac personalities, have observed their parents coping with conflicts by hurling insults at each other and, quite unconsciously, they emulate their parents' hateful behavior in their daily interactions.

If children observe parents resolving conflicts within an atmosphere of love and respect, they will be most inclined to do likewise. Few cardiac personalities have been fortunate enough to have this precious experience. Clinicians who have worked with cardiac personalities daily hear comments like the following: "Every time I yell at my wife, sooner or later I think of my father yelling at my mother. I never liked hearing my father yell at my mother, but I guess I still feel forced to copy him." "I learned from my mother that all men are wimps. That's why I can't really love my husband." "My father and mother encouraged me to be like them and tell people off when they are bothersome."

Also of crucial importance in the formation of a hostile orientation to the world is how valued the child feels in his or her day-to-day interactions with both parents. Many cardiac personalities describe their childhoods as one where they were loved conditionally. As we know, when children are loved only under certain conditions, the normal maturational process is frustrated and the child feels an inner rage.

> Rhoda, age 54, asked her physician for a referral for psychotherapy because she found herself continually in a rage. She pointed out to her physician that she was "feuding and fighting" all of her life. In her therapy she told her therapist that one of the reasons she was very full of rage as a child was because she was "always forced to be in a submissive position." Unless she complied with the edicts of her authoritarian parents, she was criticized and felt very unloved.

When children feel they must conform to arbitrary rules and regulations, they not only feel frustrated and unloved, but they begin to feel inferior (Saul 1976). They reason that what comes naturally to them seems unacceptable to their parents; consequently there must be something wrong with them.

> Sam, a man 65 years old, was the son of a football coach. His father behaved like a football coach with Sam and pressured him to play football often and play it aggressively. Annoyed with and intimidated by his father's bombastic attitude, Sam retreated to reading and other intellectual

pursuits. Inasmuch as his father was very critical of Sam's intellectual interests, Sam grew up feeling very inadequate and inferior. In his therapy with a male therapist, Sam constantly worried about being thrown out of therapy "for not talking about the right things," thus recapitulating with the therapist what he experienced with his father.

Hostility in the Therapeutic Situation

Inasmuch as cardiac personalities have difficulty experiencing most feelings except rage, of which they harbor a great deal, and because they often do not know what to do with their rage when they feel it, these behaviors inevitably become issues which confront the therapist when cardiac personalities enter therapy. Alexithymia, direct hostility, masochism, passive-aggressive behavior, depression, and turning hostility against the self are expressed in the patient's transference reactions and resistances and also affect the therapist's countertransference responses.

Transference Reactions

One of the major difficulties which therapists have in coping with cardiac personalities' behavior in the therapeutic situation is that these patients intellectualize a great deal; inasmuch as these patients are quite adept at analyzing others, they find it an onerous task to spontaneously experience and discuss their own emotions. Further, directing these patients, cajoling them, or persuading them to emote usually compounds their resistances.

With many cardiac personalities, the therapist has to cope with their intellectual, nonemotive response with much understanding, acceptance, and empathy. Otherwise the patient will feel attacked, criticized, and/or misunderstood, all of which can precipitate a premature termination of treatment.

> Tina, a single woman of 36 years, was in treatment because she had difficulty sustaining relationships with men. Always worried that she would be rejected by men, on dates she would become "tongue-tied" and say next to nothing. After a while men rejected her, feeling rejected themselves.

> Although Tina was suffering enormously, feeling depressed, physically ill, and occasionally had suicidal thoughts, in the treatment situation she was affectless and silent most of the time. When her male therapist encouraged her to talk, Tina became even more silent. When the therapist said that she was recapitulating with him what she did on dates—ignoring the therapist—Tina became even more self-conscious and silent. Eventually the therapist's impatience induced Tina to leave treatment.

In dealing with an affectless transference, therapists who work with cardiac personalities cannot rely on the usual procedure of waiting for the client to emote. As has been indicated, therapists do not help their patients very much when they admonish them to emote. What cardiac personalities need is respect for their affectless transference and empathy for their suffering.

> When Tina, in the above case, went to see another therapist, a woman, the therapist told Tina that she thought Tina was suffering a great deal. Later, she made comments about

Tina's tragic past, how dangerous it was for Tina to speak her mind, and how alone Tina must feel. As Tina was emotionally fed and well-mothered, like a loved child she began to feel more enthusiastic about her therapy and her therapist. Feeling more hopeful about her life, her symptoms diminished.

It would appear that the cardiac patient's lack of affect may be compared to the lack of appetite which many emotionally starved children feel. If forced to eat, the children will balk. If respected and accepted as they are and shown empathy for their emotional state, these children begin to feel less emotionally constricted and start to react more spontaneously. So too with the cardiac patient; if accepted as he or she is, and symbolically mothered, this patient, like Tina, moves ahead.

Cardiac personalities often form a transference that combines passive-aggressive features with masochism. In a subtle way the patient provokes the therapist by constantly suffering but is not able to acknowledge his or her hostility nor the satisfaction derived from the suffering. It is important for the therapist to realize that both the passive-aggressive behavior and the masochism are attempts to ward off direct expressions of rage.

In helping cardiac personalities to release the rage that lurks behind their maladaptive defenses of masochism and passive-aggressiveness, the clinician has to be very gentle. To confront these patients with the fact that they are defending themselves against feeling aggression is usually met with denial. Similarly, if their provocativeness is noted, they also become very defensive.

What does yield some therapeutic movement is working

with the patient's masochism. However, the clinician has to be aware that the patient derives pleasure from suffering. Therefore, he or she should discuss the patient's masochism in a neutral manner without indulging the patient. One helpful way, for example, is when the therapist comments, "I've noticed that you suffer a great deal. How did your parents respond to your suffering?" Patients usually react in one of two ways: either they point out that their parents did not notice their suffering and with some help can begin to feel and talk about their resentments, or, more sophisticated patients may be able to recall the satisfaction they derived when as children they were able to get a sympathetic response from parents and family members for their suffering. Often some patients can be helped to see how they recapitulate similar masochistic displays in the present which they displayed in their childhoods.

> Upton, a man of 58 years, was referred for psychotherapy after he had bypass surgery. Although the surgery was successful, Upton consistently behaved in a hypochondriatic way, causing his male therapist to worry constantly that Upton was getting ready to have another heart attack. In every session Upton obsessively described pains and aches in the area of his heart and, regardless of what the therapist said or did not say, Upton continued having his masochistic orgies.

> When the therapist realized that Upton was getting quite a bit of satisfaction tormenting him with his symptoms, he decided to work with Upton's masochism. He told Upton he realized that Upton had been suffering a lot and wondered how his wife was feeling as she noted all of his suffering. Without much thought, Upton declared, "By God, it's the

only time she takes notice of me!" He went on to say that it was one of the few things he could feel free to show his wife and remembered it was one of the few ways he could get his parents' attention.

After Upton talked about the "hidden pleasure" he derived from "being sick and showing it off," the therapist asked Upton if perhaps it was the only way he could get the therapist's attention and concern. With some help, Upton was able to acknowledge that it was the only way he could get anybody's care and concern. The more Upton could talk about the fact that being sick was the only way to have a caring relationship with someone, the more he could have a feeling relationship with the therapist and discuss an assortment of real feelings and real conflicts. With this the hypochondriasis subsided considerably.

A fairly frequent happenstance, occurring usually around the middle of therapy with cardiac personalities, is in the transference when they turn the therapist into a self-sufficient person who has a very good life, much better than the patient has ever had. By so doing, the patient makes the therapist into an ego ideal who is an embodiment of what the patient would like to be. Because the therapist "has it all" and the patient feels so deprived in contrast to the therapist, the latter becomes the recipient of much of the patient's hatred.

Victoria, a woman in her mid-fifties, had two bypasses. While involved in a rehabilitation program, one of her co-patients in her support group "convinced" Victoria to go into psychotherapy. Although Victoria's treatment went quite smoothly for the first few months, when her female therapist advised her that she was going on a 3-week vacation, Victoria became enraged.

Victoria spent several sessions telling her therapist what "an inconsiderate bitch" the therapist was. Furthermore, Victoria wondered how come the therapist was permitted to be a clinician inasmuch as she was "so narcissistic and insensitive to the needs of others."

While ranting about the therapist's "easy life," Victoria proposed that they switch places and take on the other's life. "Then you'd know what suffering really is and I'd know what the good life really is. It'd be a good deal," said Victoria wryly.

Because the therapist did not retaliate or censure the patient, eventually Victoria was able to examine herself. She talked about how she always felt like "a have not" in her own family and how much better off her older brother and sister were. After her hostility was fully discharged, Victoria could face for the first time in her life her acute dependency yearnings.

Hostile Resistances

For therapy to be effective, the patient should more and more be able to discuss with the therapist everything that is on his or her mind and concomitantly experience a wide range of feelings while doing so. As has been demonstrated, cardiac personalities have a difficult time achieving this goal. To ward off the anxiety which evolves if they face the true facts of their lives, and to spare the therapist hearing the hostility which is always within them, cardiac personalities can become preoccupied with everyday trivia and try to have extensive discussions with the therapist about the trivia.

As the therapist hears in session after session minutiae such as brushing teeth, buying groceries, or naps taken, it is easy to feel bored and to ignore the content of the patient's sessions. If this continues, sooner or later the patient and/or the therapist find some justification to end the treatment prematurely because both feel uninvolved in it.

One way out of this possible stalemate is for the therapist to show some interest and to ask some questions about the patient's mundane affairs. Many patients are shocked to find somebody interested in what is usually ignored in their daily interactions. But, when they feel the therapist's interest is genuine, they can become much more responsive to the treatment.

> Walter, age 62, was in treatment for a variety of reasons. He had acute sexual problems, was depressed much of the time, could not succeed in his work as an accountant, felt very unappreciated by his wife and children, and had no close relationships. In addition he suffered from many psychosomatic problems including hypertension.

> After reading off in his first session with his male therapist a list of his problems, Walter then spent each of his following therapy sessions reviewing his monotonous week. He told the therapist what time he awoke in the morning, how long he spent in the shower, what he had for breakfast, how long he waited for the subway, and so forth. He described his work and the rest of his life in the same dreary manner.

> After about 4 months of weekly therapy, when the therapist found himself becoming quite sleepy in almost every session and realized he was ignoring almost everything Walter was

saying, he began to study his own reactions much more carefully. One of the therapist's hypotheses about the stalemate was the possibility that Walter unconsciously wanted to be ignored and that a closer involvement between therapist and patient might stir up too much anxiety for Walter.

Experiencing much less guilt about feeling bored, because he could accept with more conviction that Walter wanted a great deal of distance, the therapist attempted an experiment. He reasoned as follows: "If Walter wants distance and to keep the status quo, any interest on my part would upset him. If in fact he gets upset with me when I show interest in him, that would be great because it would be the first time he's shown some affect."

Therefore the next time Walter talked about the time he woke up and took a shower, the therapist took the opportunity to ask him questions about his showering habits. Was it daily? What temperature water did he like best? What kind of soap was used?

At first, Walter dismissed the therapist's questions. However, when the therapist asked Walter how come he was dismissing his questions, Walter at first became withdrawn. A little later in the session he became exasperated. Near the end of the session he became very angry at the therapist for "asking stupid questions," and he questioned the therapist's sincerity.

As Walter could express more anger toward the therapist, both patient and therapist began to find the treatment sessions much more interesting. After berating the therapist, Walter went on to attack his own parents and sister for their neglect of him. As he brought out a lot of rage toward family members, and others too, he could see how terrified he had been of his own aggression. However, because he could eventually sense the therapist's interest in him, Walter was able to examine his hostility in more depth and breadth and in a safer environment. After one-and-one-half years of therapy, Walter was a much more communicative man who was suffering much less from depression and psychosomatic difficulties. Slowly he was turning his hostility into normal assertiveness.

Another form of resistance seen quite frequently in cardiac personalities is gossiping about the therapist in negative terms. The reason negative gossip is used frequently by cardiac personalities is that it affords them an outlet for their aggression, but the object of the aggression, in this case the therapist, does not have to be faced directly. By not having to confront the therapist, the patient does not have to worry as much about retaliation.

Although it may be considered an indirect form of gossip, perhaps a sublimatory expression, cardiac personalities often seek out consultations with other therapists to discuss their criticisms of their current helper. In that way they hope to find an expert to reinforce their own hostility. (Occasionally they want the therapist they consult to talk them out of their resentment.)

What my colleagues and I have noted about the gossiping of cardiac personalities is that sooner or later (but usually sooner), their negative remarks about the therapist get back to him or her. This should not surprise us. Cardiac personalities, though harboring much hostility, usually feel guilty about it and unconsciously seek punishment for it. Though fearful of the therapist's possible counterattacks, in many ways they believe they deserve and need them in order to wipe away their guilt. Therefore, cardiac personalities can "arrange" to gossip in a manner which brings the news to the therapist. Or, in some cases, they can confess directly to the therapist that they have been gossiping.

When dealing with their patients' gossiping about them, it is imperative for clinicians to monitor their own narcissism and anger and keep in mind that expressions of hostility from the patient, particularly indirect forms like gossiping, emanate from the patient's feelings of threat, vulnerability, envy, and inferiority. Otherwise, patient and therapist can get into a hostile power struggle about the meaning of the patient's activities.

> Yolanda, age 58, was in treatment at a low-cost mental health clinic. In addition to her stormy marriage of 30 years, she wanted help for her frequent altercations with her children and grandchildren. Also, she found her job as a salesperson in a bookstore very trying. At times her anxiety turned into somatic problems such as headaches, stomachaches, and breathlessness.

> After being in treatment for about 6 months, during which time she alternated between finding fault with the therapy and the therapist, and praising her female therapist, Yolanda began making negative remarks in the waiting room of the clinic about her therapist. She gossiped to other patients about the therapist and approached other clinicians in the waiting room and asked them what she should do about her therapist who wasn't helping her.

> After the therapist received about five or six reports that Yolanda had been complaining and criticizing her, the

therapist shared this information with her. Yolanda, despite the reliability of the witnesses, denied that she had been gossiping. The therapist, having felt derided for several weeks and now manipulated in the present, asked Yolanda why she could not tell her the truth. The accusation only made Yolanda more defensive and a few weeks later she quit treatment.

When a patient finds it difficult to tell the therapist the truth, the therapist's first job is to try to make it safer for the patient to do so. In Yolanda's case, it would have been helpful if the therapist had said something like, "I'm not making it safe enough for you here. It's difficult to share your criticisms about me with me." This might have helped Yolanda voice her complaints, and with her hostility accepted by the therapist, she might have been able eventually to face the feeling of vulnerability, inferiority, envy, and anxiety that helped spark her wish to gossip about the therapist.

Another resistance of cardiac personalities which emerges frequently during hostile phases of treatment are attempts by the patient to engage the therapist in discussion about the advantages and disadvantages of psychotherapy. Usually the patient is not examining what he or she feels but unconsciously is trying to engage the therapist in an argument.

Whenever any patient wants to argue the merits of therapy with the therapist, the patient is usually feeling very ambivalent about the therapy. To try to convince the patient that being in therapy will be of help will only lead to more arguments. And, if the therapist feels disillusioned and tells the patient that maybe ending treatment is a reasonable idea, the patient will probably oppose that idea as well! Ambivalent patients are always championing "the other side."

   The best way to help patients resolve their ambivalence is by never arguing with them and never trying to convince them. Rather, patients are best helped when the therapist shares with them his or her impression that their patients are having a real struggle with the therapy and having mixed feelings about being a patient. Although patients will continue to make attempts to argue, if the therapist keeps the focus on the patient's ambivalent feelings about treatment, eventually most patients will probably be able to discuss openly their struggle about being in treatment.

> Zangwill, a man in his mid-seventies, was referred to psychotherapy by his physician because of extreme anxiety about his cardiac symptoms which, the physician believed, were exacerbated by his anxiety.
>
> After no more than three or four treatment sessions with his male therapist, Zangwill began to question the advisability of his being in treatment. He did not discuss his ambivalence, just talked about mental arguments he was having with the authors of books on emotional problems and psychotherapy. As he presented these arguments in his therapy sessions, Zangwill sounded like a lawyer turning the authors into adversaries.
>
> When the therapist said little but listened attentively, Zangwill slowly but surely tried to draw the therapist into these arguments. Though the therapist was tempted to try to refute some of his patient's statements, he managed to stay out of the fight. When the therapist told Zangwill after 3 months of therapy that he thought Zangwill had mixed feelings about being his patient, Zangwill ignored the statement but instead kept on obsessing about how "many people can manage without a therapist" and that "many therapists

were worse off than their patients." During the fourth month of therapy after Zangwill mentioned that a lot of therapists were unethical and then asked the therapist, "Don't you agree?" the therapist responded by saying, "I think you'd rather argue with me about therapy than talk about your own mixed feelings." This statement seemed to help Zangwill and he shifted his presentation.

Zangwill began openly to attack the therapist and told him that he was unethical and making money out of an "inexact science." He also told the therapist that he believed that the therapist had "serious psychological problems" but that he was "scared to admit it."

During the sixth month of treatment, after Zangwill had repeatedly attacked and demeaned the therapist, Zangwill began to change his tune. He told the therapist in a noncritical manner that he was surprised that the therapist "didn't hit back." When the therapist said, "It's more important to understand your anger than anything else," Zangwill responded by saying "You know, I'm beginning to like you."

For the next several months, Zangwill was able to explore with the therapist his strong feelings of weakness, inferiority, and vulnerability that were major factors accounting for his vituperative outbursts. Slowly he began to assert himself in a much more constructive way and with very limited guile.

Countertransference Reactions to Hostile Transference Responses

Inasmuch as many cardiac personalities use their hostility in the treatment situation to block any sense of being party to a close relationship, it is not difficult for the therapist to feel lonely and unimportant as he or she attempts to involve these patients in a therapeutic relationship.

In his paper "Aloneness in the Countertransference," Roy Schafer (1995) has described a type of patient who induces feelings of insignificance and loneliness in the therapist. These patients, as Schafer portrays them, sound remarkably similar to cardiac personalities.

> [These patients] have had extremely painful and infuriating experiences of being the captives of harsh introjects.... They feel that they have lived their lives in enemy territory or as though they were standing before burning bushes into which they do not dare to look. Therefore, anything that resembles fraternizing with the [therapist], such as eye contact, informality, or familiarity, remains out of the question....

> Frightened as they are, yet when described along another line, they may be characterized differently, specifically as occupying positions of omnipotence. They are omnipotent in a limited universe: in one way, rulers of all they survey; in another way rulers of all they overlook or banish. What they can't see can't hurt them—so they hope! And in its more benevolent aspects, what they don't see can't hurt their objects either. [pp. 508-509]

When therapists feel isolated, alone, and not useful in the treatment relationship, they are often inclined to take measures to bolster their self-esteem and tend to become more active in the therapy sessions. It is not always easy for clinicians to remember that cardiac personalities become even more resistant when they have to face a therapist who is trying hard to appear intelligent, competent, and useful.

If therapists find they are very active in the therapy sessions, it is usually a clue to them that they are feeling unimportant and trying too hard to make themselves important. Feeling unimportant, of course, is one of the main problems of cardiac personalities and they are not going to be too indulgent of the therapist's unresolved conflicts in this area. They are the ones who want to feel important and they will fight it out, directly or indirectly, with the therapist who they experience as untherapeutically overactive.

When therapists realize they are being overactive, largely because they want to repair their damaged self-esteem, they should take some time to find out why the patient's rejection of them is bothersome and threatening. Secondly, they should attempt to get in touch with who the patient represents to them. Is it a rivalrous sibling? An ambivalent parent? Thirdly, it is often helpful to therapists when they realize they are talking too much to try their best to keep quiet in the sessions and see just what they feel. This will usually help them define their countertransference issues in more detail and dynamic terms.

> Zenia, age 39, was in treatment with Dr. C. for several reasons. She was unhappy in her job as a guidance counselor, finding the work unstimulating and ungratifying. She experienced her husband as very boring and, in addition, her two children, a daughter of 8 and a son of 6, were hard for her to manage. When she found herself having insomnia, gastrointestinal problems, hypertension, and other physical symptoms, she sought therapy.

For the first 2 months of her twice a week therapy, Zenia seemed to be positively involved in it. She talked openly about her marital and work difficulties and seemed to get quite a bit of relief from doing so. She also reported that her somatic symptoms had diminished.

After having told Dr. C. in the third month of therapy that she was "getting something out of this," Zenia's manner and tone changed rather dramatically. Instead of discussing her interpersonal problems, in a dull manner she described in detail her somatic difficulties. When this became repetitive, Dr. C. made continued interpretations of Zenia's resistance to discussing her problems about her family and job. Although Zenia listened to these interpretations, she responded with more detailed renditions of her bodily problems and went into them in still more detail.

Observing that Zenia was unresponsive to his interventions, Dr. C. decided to make interpretations regarding Zenia's transference resistances. As could have been predicted, Zenia became more involved in discussing bodily problems, and, in fact, felt more aches and pains.

Dr. C., recognizing the stalemate in his work with Zenia, consulted a colleague. From his consultation, he realized that Zenia did progress when he attentively listened to her during the first couple of months of treatment. Dr. C. further recognized that it made Zenia feel very vulnerable to acknowledge her progress in therapy and her gratitude to Dr. C. That was why she moved away from him. Dr. C. became aware that if he were going to help Zenia, he had to respect her resistances more, not try so hard to impress her with his knowledge, and not confront her so often with her recalcitrance.

As Dr. C. remained quieter and more attentive, asking only occasional questions about Zenia's aches and pains, she started to become much more revealing and more related to Dr. C.

When therapists deal with cardiac personalities, most of whom are harboring much hostility, it is not surprising to find them unleashing some of their own hostility in the sessions. Therapists, like their patients, can feel frustrated, humiliated, and unloved. As we have seen throughout this chapter, hatred is a response to these emotional conditions. Consequently, when acting hostilely toward their patients, therapists need to do for themselves what they try to do for their patients, that is, get in touch with the vulnerable feelings that have provoked their hatred.

> Yussel, a 49-year-old man, was in treatment because he had severe marital difficulties. In his therapy with Dr. D., a female therapist, he spent most of his sessions attacking his wife. He severely criticized her for being a poor lover, homemaker, mother, and friend. As far as Yussel was concerned, his wife could do nothing right.

> Whenever Dr. D. tried to help Yussel look at himself and see what his role was in his marital difficulties, he became very defensive and started to treat Dr. D. with a lot of contempt. Confronted with his contempt toward both his wife and therapist, Yussel threatened to quit therapy altogether.

> Dr. D. found herself feeling progressively more angry with Yussel. In one session she could feel her voice rising and her face reddening. Of course, with some pleasure, Yussel noticed this reaction of his therapist, and demeaned her again.

Eventually Dr. D. began to confront her own hostility. She learned that she was feeling consistently wiped out by her patient and wanted to "return the favor." The more Dr. D. could recognize how insignificant she felt next to Yussel, the more she could feel how terribly insignificant Yussel felt next to her.

With her increased self-awareness, Dr. D. could listen more and talk less in her sessions with Yussel. When she intervened she spoke of how alone Yussel felt in his marriage, how disappointed he was with his wife, and how terribly misunderstood he had felt by the women in his life, including Dr. D.

As Yussel felt better understood and less attacked by Dr. D., he began to try to understand himself and his wife more, and he was less hostile toward everyone in his social orbit.

Virtually every researcher who has investigated the emotional life of cardiac personalities recognized how much hostility is present in them and how pervasive it is. What is sometimes insufficiently appreciated by therapists who work with patients with cardiovascular disorders is that their hostility is a response to feeling unloved, unappreciated, and misunderstood. As the psychiatrist Alexander Lowen (1988) has stated in his book *Love, Sex, and Your Heart*, "Hate can be described as love turned cold. The process is not quick; for love to freeze, it requires repeated disappointments" (p. 14).

What is important for clinicians to keep in mind is that when hatred is met with a hostile reaction, the patient has no recourse but to withdraw from the relationship. On the other hand, if the patient's rage is discussed in an accepting atmosphere, he or she begins to face his or her tremendous difficulties with dependency feelings and problems of loving and being loved—the focus of our next chapter.

6

From
Pseudo-independence
to Healthy
Dependency

In the preceding chapters we have tried to understand how the defenses of omnipotence and hostility are utilized by cardiac personalities to protect themselves from feeling vulnerable, anxious, envious, panicky, and a host of other painful emotional states. What we would like to focus on now is what it is that gives rise to the cardiac personalities' defenses of omnipotence and hostility: namely, frustrated dependency.

As we have observed in previous chapters, cardiac personalities tend to suffer a loss of love in early childhood which often leaves them "broken-hearted." The pain and anguish which results from the "heartless" behavior they have frequently had to endure from others forces them to be pseudo-independent, grandiose, affectless much of the time, and hostile a good part of the time. Alexander Lowen (1988) has described how those destined to suffer from heart disease and/or a heart attack repress the pain that evolves from heartless love by armoring themselves, that is, by rigidifying the muscles in their chest walls. He points out:

> This rigidification restricts and limits breathing,
> movement, and feeling, imposing a continuous
> stress on the body and the heart. It is the existence
> of this sort of stress that predisposes so many
> people to heart disease. [p. 107]

As we study the problems with dependency which cardiac personalities experience, we will see that because they cannot trust themselves to love or be loved (Erikson 1950), their marriages are compromised, their work lives fill them with enormous obligations and pressures, and their day-to-day interactions are often ungratifying. Because they are afraid to love, their hearts cannot be completely healthy.

In *Treating Type A Behavior and Your Heart*, Friedman and Roseman (1984) came to the conclusion that a lack of love is largely responsible for Type A behavior. "We now believe," they state, "that one of the most important influences fostering insecurity is the failure of the Type A person in his infancy and early childhood to receive unconditional love, affection, and encouragement from one or both parents" (p. 45). In this situation, the Type A individual has but one choice: to engage in "a continuous struggle, an unremitting attempt to accomplish or achieve more and more in less and less time" (p. 31).

James Lynch (1977), in *The Broken Heart*, refers to several studies that show a marked rise in death rates during the first 6 months following the loss of a loved one. In 75 percent of the cases studied, death was caused by coronary artery disease, a statistic that tends to document the damaging effect the loss of love can have on the heart.

A study conducted by Stewart Wolff and Helen Goodell

(1962) of the inhabitants of Roseto, Pennsylvania, demonstrated that the instability of interpersonal relationships has a harmful effect on the heart. Roseto, up until the 1940s, was a town of 1,600 people, mostly Italian, that had only one-third as many heart attacks as people in surrounding communities, despite the fact that their diets and cholesterol levels were about the same. What seemed to protect these people against heart disease was their quality of life. The family was the focus of daily life and the inhabitants retained the customs and traditions from their homeland. However, the town underwent a tremendous change over two decades. Industry moved in, real estate prospered, and the family was no longer the center of life. By 1960, the vital statistics of health and disease showed that Roseto had become similar to its surrounding communities, with the incidence of heart disease and heart attacks no different from theirs.

As we have noted, the family stability which initially characterized Roseto with its consistent gratification of dependency wishes and the constant mutual expression of love does not exist too much in our current society. Instead, we have much marital instability and parent–child conflict. With limited gratification of mutual love in much of our society, it should not surprise us as we noted in Chapter 1 that heart disease is the Number One killer of men and women in the United States.

How we feel about mutual dependency as adults is very much affected by the mutuality, or lack thereof, which transpired between our parents and ourselves during the first years of our lives. As we reached out for closeness as infants, if the response was tender, loving, and caring, it filled us with pleasure. If nothing disturbed the loving relationship, we became "light-hearted," happy children and began to believe that human transactions are for the most part joyous. If, on the other hand, our parents were ambivalent, unavailable, or inconsistent, we felt pain and panic. Although we did not recognize it, the pain and panic was an introduction to heart problems.

Researchers have demonstrated that when a child experiences a loss of love from an important person or persons, the blood that had been sent to the surface of the body is suddenly withdrawn to the interior. The heart is now engorged with more blood than it can expel. The pressure builds and the heart feels as if it would burst because the whole body goes into a state of contraction. The unloved child or inconsistently loved child is a real candidate for heart disease because the bodily pressure that has just been described is the opposite of the state of expansion which love produces (Lowen 1988).

In his studies of early childhood, Erik Erikson (1950) demonstrated that if the child's dependency wishes are gratified consistently and lovingly, not only does the child trust the world, but he or she develops an inner certainty and a hopefulness about life. It is of interest that many of the writers on heart disease who focus on emotional factors concur that the cardiac personality is one with limited hope (Cousins 1983, Lowen 1988, Lynch 1977). States Lowen (1988): "One can tolerate being trapped in a painful situation as long as there is some hope in the heart. There is a saying that there is hope as long as the heart beats. This implies that cardiac arrest is equivalent to a loss of hope" (pp. 139–140).

Dependency Conflicts in Love and Marriage

In order for a love relationship to sustain itself warmly and positively, the two individuals must be able to feel quite relaxed about depending on each other. This is not usually true with cardiac personalities. They view their partners with suspicion, concerned that they will be betrayed at any moment. It is not that they do not have loving feelings toward their mates. Rather, they are in a continual state of ambivalence: wanting to love and be loved, worried that it won't be forthcoming, and upset that there is always tension in the relationship which, of course, causes stress and is dangerous to the heart.

When a man or woman cannot fully trust the partner, sex almost always becomes a problem. In order to enjoy sex, both partners must feel the freedom to regress and temporarily symbiose with each other. If either partner has had difficulty with being held, touched, and so forth, there will be a resistance to penetrating and being penetrated. Then, sex will activate anxiety and resentment.

Abramov (1976) compared the sexual lives of 100 women, aged 40 to 60, who were hospitalized for an acute myocardial infarction, with a control group of 100 women of the same ages who were hospitalized for other illnesses. Sexual dissatisfaction was found among 65 percent of the coronary patients compared to 24 percent of the control group. These statistics seem to indicate that a lack of sexual satisfaction could be considered a risk factor for heart disease in women.

In a study of male sexual dysfunction, Wahrer and Burchell (1980) examined 131 men, aged 31 to 86, who all been hospitalized for heart attacks; two-thirds were found to have experienced significant sexual problems prior to the attack. Sixty-four percent of the subjects were impotent, 28 percent had experienced a 50 percent decrease in sexual frequency, and 8 percent suffered from premature ejaculation.

Warren, age 48, was in intensive therapy, seeing his female therapist three times a week. A competent lawyer, Warren was frequently impotent with his wife and often had limited desire to even embrace her. In addition to his sexual difficulties, Warren suffered from migraine headaches, asthma, gastrointestinal problems, and hypertension.

In therapy, when Warren discussed his relationship with his wife, his emotions were blunted. As this was worked on in treatment, Warren discovered how much he resented his wife "for being so unreliable." Though his wife was quite loyal and devoted, Warren often had "a sinking feeling that she would yell and scream" at him for little provocation. Examining his suspicions, Warren was able to see how much he related to his wife as if she were the tyrannical mother of his past and he were her intimidated son. Feeling like a young son with a mother, it was quite clear why having sex with his wife was uncomfortable.

Frequently, a cardiac personality who is frightened of his or her own dependency yearnings will marry a spouse who is very dependent. The cardiac personality can deny wishes to be taken care of and vicariously be indulged while ministering to the partner. One of the difficulties with this type of arrangement is that the giver (usually the cardiac personality) resents all of the demands and feels trapped in an ungratifying relationship.

A woman in her late thirties, Vivian was in treatment at a mental health center because of her sexual problems. In her therapy with a male, Vivian took all of the responsibility for her lack of sexual satisfaction in her marriage and contended that her husband was a good lover.

As the therapy moved on, it became apparent to Vivian and her therapist that much of her *modus vivendi* was one of self-sacrificing. Vivian anticipated all of her husband's demands and catered to him incessantly. In addition, the idea of having wishes of her own and having them gratified seemed foreign to her. She behaved similarly with her young daughter as well.

After she had been in treatment about 6 months, Vivian had a dream in which she was throwing shoes at her husband and while doing so was yelling and cursing at him. With the therapist's help, Vivian could eventually acknowledge how much she wanted to hit and kick her husband "for being a big baby." Although it was a major breakthrough to feel her rage, it took over a year and a half of twice weekly therapy for Vivian to see that she was the one who wanted to be a "big baby" but was busy fighting the idea.

As we have observed in previous chapters, a chronic marital complaint is really an unconscious wish. One of the chronic marital complaints that is frequently observed among cardiac personalities is the strong conviction that they are working overtime taking care of the needs and wishes of their partners, while they, the mistreated, are suffering and deprived. Although there is a great deal of reality in these chronic marital complaints, what is important for the clinician to keep in mind is that the complaint protects and gratifies the complainer. He or she is frightened to say, "I would like you to give me..." Rather, he or she would prefer to say, "You are unkind. You give me next to nothing." In this way, the dependency wishes are denied and the complainer can discharge all kinds of hostility with some impunity.

Usher, a man in his sixties, was being seen at a family agency for marital counseling. The treatment was conjoint; that is, Usher and his wife were seen together by one therapist.

In many sessions, Usher complained that his wife was unavailable to help him with chores around the house, did not respond positively to his sexual overtures, and never complimented him. Furthermore, she did not seem to appreciate the fact that he was a very competent breadwinner.

In the marriage counseling sessions, Usher's wife Sarah listened attentively to Usher's complaints, but every time she tried to say something, Usher stopped her and went on to complain some more. Finally, the female therapist intervened to point this out. When Usher relented and said to Sarah, "Okay, okay, what do you want to say?" Sarah stated, "I really want to try to be different. I'll help you with the chores more than I do. I'll try to be more responsive sexually. I really appreciate you. You are an excellent husband." After a moment of silence, Usher bellowed, "I don't believe you. You are a liar. You don't want to give me a damn thing."

It took Usher many months to see how he was his own worst enemy and really was very frightened to be dependent on Sarah in any way.

Not until the cardiac personality is able to gratify his or her dependency wishes without feeling like a disturbed and vulnerable child will he or she be able to enjoy an intimate, loving relationship. To be able to enjoy and love a mate, the partner must be accepted and understood as he or she is. Most cardiac personalities are unwittingly busy making the mate a depriving parent of their past. This distortion accounts in many ways for their marital unhappiness.

Dependency Problems at Work

Any sensitive administrator or executive is very aware of the reality that early dependency problems among their staff becomes recapitulated in the work situation. Most supervisors and executives are experienced as parental figures and are often the recipient of feelings and fantasies that those under them have not resolved toward their parents.

A very common problem of workers is they make each other siblings and compete for the love of the boss. Cardiac personalities, who have often felt like the scapegoat in their original families, become unduly hurt and angry when their colleagues receive praise and attention from the boss. This is frequently experienced by them as if they are the despised scapegoat and the colleague is the loved sibling. The hurt and anger is often held within, and heart problems can be a consequence.

> Terry, a 52-year-old high school teacher, had suffered a heart attack. As part of her rehabilitation, psychotherapy was recommended.
>
> In her therapy, she told her male therapist that every time the principal of the high school just smiled at a colleague of hers, Terry could feel her "heart burn."
>
> As Terry and her therapist examined her life, it became apparent that she was still feeling very betrayed by both of

her parents who seemed to favor her older brother when she was a child. Unable to resolve her deep hurt and anger toward her parents, Terry recapitulated her conflicts in work situations. She labored very hard to enlist the love of those in authority and competed intensely for their love with all of her colleagues.

Interestingly, Terry felt her conflicts much more in the work situation than at home with her husband and children. When her therapist and she investigated this, Terry commented, "At home, I know I'm the only wife and the only mother. At work, I have to share the attention and it reminds me too much of being at home with my parents and brother."

Though we have referred several times to the notion that cardiac personalities are frequently workaholics, we have not sufficiently demonstrated how their dependency problems enter into the picture. What seems to happen when one is addicted to work is the same phenomenon that occurs in every addiction. Just as the alcoholic takes a drink rather than relying on the love of another human being, the workaholic substitutes work for human contact. Not able to permit themselves to be dependent on a spouse or lover, workaholics become overly attached to work.

What is often overlooked in assessing the dynamics of work addicts is, because they put in so much time and energy into their work, they inevitably resent the workplace, despite being symbiotically tied to it. Workaholics, in effect, are like husbands and wives who can't feel the freedom to be autonomous. Consequently, they are devoted mates, but resent their many obligations, which, it is important to emphasize, are for the most part self-imposed.

In *The Healing Heart*, Norman Cousins (1983) points out

that "people who feel locked into obligations that they would rather set aside are candidates for sudden and severe disease" (p. 36). Cousins suffered a heart attack at home after a return from "a hectic trip to the East Coast just before Christmas time" (p. 35). He was very resentful of having to take another trip to the Southeast in a few days, which he thought might be too difficult to cancel. Feeling very pressured to fulfill his next assignment, but resenting it, Cousins was in a state of intense indecision. The next day he had a heart attack.

For cardiac personalities, expending excessive energy in the work situation is equivalent to knocking themselves out for parents whose love they desperately crave. However, cardiac personalities, after a while, become exasperated with how much they have to do and how much time it takes for them to do it. Working hard to procure equivalents of love becomes a very tedious job!

Considering how much workaholics resent the many burdens the job places on them, having a heart attack, and lying still for a long while may be viewed as an unconscious attempt "to get away from it all." Friedman and Rosenman (1984) learned that over half of the men in their study who had heart attacks not only expected to have one but "yearned" for it. One patient enjoyed having no responsibilities while being taken care of by pretty nurses. Another averred that having a heart attack gave him permission to retire from work.

With regard to the unconscious motives involved in a heart attack, Alexander Lowen (1988) has suggested the following:

> For some people, a heart attack may seem the only way to escape the stresses and strains of a pressured

> existence. Some then go on to make the kind of
> changes in their lives that might have prevented the
> attack. Is there in such people a need to suffer,
> stemming perhaps from some deep sense of guilt, so
> that only after they have paid a price are they free to
> make some positive moves in their lives? [p.160]

The guilt that Lowen refers to comes from the patient's hostility. However, what is important to keep in mind is that the hostility is a response to frustrated dependency wishes. Not able to derive love from overworking, the cardiac personality is furious about the deprivations and frustrations which are endured daily. To feel them consciously, to express them directly, stirs up excessive guilt. Therefore, to have a heart attack, which forces the person to stop working, seems like "a logical choice."

In *Staying the Course: The Emotional and Social Lives of Men Who do Well at Work*, Robert Weiss (1990) points out how work stress makes many men extremely difficult to live with because they are so preoccupied and distant from their mates and children. Feeling stressed at work and not too well tolerated at home make for longer-term consequences such as "depression, burnout, and somatic disorders." Weiss, like other writers, views physical distress as an unconscious plea to get away from work.

As we have noted in earlier chapters, most cardiac personalities have a strong desire to renounce their dependency wishes and become "defensively autonomous" (Levant 1995). They find it difficult to share with mates and peers how difficult work is and "the alone feeling" becomes exacerbated until they have to express the struggle bodily.

Stan, 52 years old, an assistant principal in a junior high school, was very devoted to his superior, to the teachers and children with whom he worked, and to the parents of the schoolchildren. He worked day and night "taking care of everybody."

Since he had a smiling face almost all the time, it shocked everybody around him when they heard that Stan was in a deep depression and had suffered a heart attack.

It took Stan many months of psychotherapy before he could face not only how resentful he was about the many demands on him but how deeply he craved for recognition that was rarely forthcoming.

Some cardiac personalities, as children, could get a response from their parents only if they provoked them. Coming from families where "children should be seen but not heard," they tend to feel in the present that the only way they can get a superior's attention is by upsetting him or her. It is very important for clinicians to keep in mind when listening to patients describing fights with the boss that their patients may be deriving a secret satisfaction in getting a rise out of the boss. Also, the patient may be enjoying turning on the therapist as he or she listens to dramatic events from the workplace.

Rhoda, age 48, was an advertising executive who sought therapy for depression, migraine headaches, and other somatic complaints. Divorced and childless, Rhoda gave much of her time and attention to her work.

What emerged quite early in her therapy with her female therapist were her repeated complaints that her male superior took her for granted. In many ways, she sounded like the rebuffed wife who was hurt that her "boss/husband" did not pay sufficient attention to her.

During Rhoda's fourth month of twice weekly therapy, she began to discuss with her therapist long and frequent arguments with her boss. The arguments focused on superficial issues but clearly induced intense emotions in the boss and Rhoda.

As the arguments were carefully investigated in therapy, and Rhoda's feelings were elicited, Rhoda, in her eighth month of therapy, stated, "He [the boss] reminds me of my father. The only way I could get the old guy to notice me was to fight with him. I guess that's what I'm doing at work with another old guy."

As we see, the workplace for the cardiac personality is usually filled with problems. Until he or she can believe that work is to be enjoyed and can begin to enjoy it consistently, cardiac problems do not have a full chance to be resolved.

Dependency in Everyday Life

In the chapter on stress, Chapter 2, we discussed at length how loneliness and social isolation contribute heavily to heart disease because of the disabling properties of stress. Because cardiac personalities are very frightened of their dependency wishes and fight their expression daily, loneliness and social isolation are inevitable.

As we have consistently pointed out, cardiac personalities want to depend on mates, friends, colleagues, and so forth.

However, they have a strong tendency to turn peers, mates, and others into figures of the past and then anticipate rejection from them. Rather than deal with the humiliation and pain of feeling rejected, if it occurs, cardiac personalities tend to shun intimacy in order to protect themselves.

Those experts who have dealt with the emotional components of heart disease (for example, Benson 1993, Chopra 1993, Cortis 1995, Cousins 1983, Flannery 1990, Ornish 1990) have all concluded that loneliness and social isolation almost always accompany heart disease. They also concur with the notion that bringing the cardiac personality into contact with other human beings will reverse heart disease.

One of the reasons that most experts have such strong conviction about helping the cardiac personality learn how to depend on others more is because there is strong empirical support for this perspective. In addition to the research we have mentioned (for example, Cousins 1989, Lynch 1985, Ornish 1990), in a recent article, "Effects of Psychosocial Interactions at a Cellular Level," Nee (1995) has been able to demonstrate conclusively in a series of studies how social isolation diminishes longevity and social intimacy prolongs it. House and colleagues (1988) found that the effect of lack of social interaction on mortality is similar to other well-established health risks, including high serum cholesterol, smoking, and high blood pressure. In the laboratory it has become abundantly clear that there is probably no organ system or homeostatic defense mechanism that is not influenced by the interaction between the social self and the somatic self.

What is very important for the mental health professional to keep in mind about this issue is the tremendous anxiety and powerful resistances that cardiac personalities experience when they merely think of increasing the quantity and quality of their social relationships. Bombarded by much suspiciousness and distrust which borders on paranoid thinking, almost every person and event that they think of confronting during the day can induce anguish for them. Yearning for contact, but terribly worried that the other person will betray them, they rarely can relax as they contemplate most forms of social interaction.

Quentin, in his late fifties, described a typical day of his to the social worker who was treating him at an outpatient treatment center of a hospital. "When I get up in the morning it's usually after a restless night. Most of the time I have nightmares with bullies chasing me, trying to steal something from me. Then when I go to the bathroom, I'm always worried that my wife or the kids did something to stop the toilet from flushing or the shower from working. Then, I'm in a rage because I'm convinced my wife forgot to buy soap.

"I worry that there's not going to be enough to eat at breakfast and while eating I'm convinced the mechanic screwed things up so I won't be able to drive the car. I'm furious while driving to work, quite sure someone is going to bang into me, and if I'm not worried about that, I'm planning who is not going to return my phone calls when I get to the office. I'm almost positive that the guy with whom I have a lunch appointment is not going to show up.

"While I'm away from my house and supposed to be busy at work in the office, I'm also wondering what my wife is planning to do to hurt me. Sometimes I picture her having an affair while I'm gone. Nothing goes right for me. I don't trust a soul. I can't depend on anyone at anytime. Sometimes I wish that I were Superman. Then I could run the whole world and the world couldn't run me down."

Although Quentin probably suffers more each day than do most cardiac personalities, his dynamics are typical of them. Learning to be given to and taken care of, Quentin is convinced that nobody will be there for him. With his dependency wishes constantly frustrated, he is in a constant rage. Overwhelmed by constant stress and never feeling certain, he fantasies himself as omnipotent, that is, a superman. As we know, the possibility of his becoming a superman is remote. Consequently, the sequence of frustrated dependency leading to hostility and omnipotence goes on many times during the course of each day.

One of the necessities in daily life is asking others for small favors. Most of us need traffic directions from time to time. We need assistance from colleagues, friends, and family to arrange a mutually convenient time for meals, meetings, and recreation. No human being can be an island for too long, but cardiac personalities often feel they must be an island unto themselves most of the time. Fearful that their requests will make them look small and weak, frightened of rejection, impelled to be omnipotent, the cardiac personality is often saying to others, both overtly and covertly, "Don't do me any favors."

> Penny, a 43-year-old married woman, was very eager to get herself a job, now that her children were older and more self-sufficient. When her therapist, a woman about her own age, observed that Penny was very reluctant to make contact with prospective employers and asked Penny about that reluctance, she learned a lot about Penny's enormous fear of dependency.

> Penny told her therapist that she could sit around the phone for hours at a time, frightened that if she asked for an

interview, she would emerge "as an obnoxious, pesty child who wants too much." What became apparent as Penny discussed her anxiety about asking for a job interview is the same inhibition that existed in many dimensions of her daily life. She was "scared" to ask a woman friend to go for a walk because she would feel "too imposing." If she thought of entertaining at her home, she worried that people would not want to come to her house. And, if they did, "they would be faking it" because she was convinced she was not well-liked. "I've learned to be self-sufficient much of the time," Penny concluded.

Discussing the theme of self-sufficiency, Offit (1995) has opined:

> [There are] people whose upbringing has taught them either the virtues or the necessity of detachment. When this is ego syntonic, or experienced as a positive quality, the person takes pride in not needing anyone. To feel possessiveness or jealousy is experienced as infantile absurdity which [they believe] every adult must outgrow as soon as possible, or be considered hopelessly juvenile. [p.28]

In order to enjoy social interaction with others, a number of personal qualities are necessary which many cardiac personalities lack. Not only must one feel a certain ease in depending on others and being depended upon, but one must be able to accept the limitations of others and be able to forgive them when they have provoked us or ignored us.

Cardiac personalities are so ready to continue their sadomasochistic relationships of their pasts that they would rather feel angry at friends and colleagues for what they cannot provide. Therefore they find it impossible to forgive because that would mean they are ready to try to renew a mutually trusting and mutually dependent relationship. Otto Kernberg (1995) relates to this issue with much eloquence:

> The capacity to forgive others is usually a sign of a mature superego, stemming from having been able to recognize aggression and ambivalence in oneself and from the related capacity to accept the ambivalence that is unavoidable in intimate relations. Authentic forgiveness is an expression of a mature sense of morality, an acceptance of the pain that comes with the loss of illusions about self and other, faith in the possibility of the recovery of trust, the possibility that love will be recreated and maintained in spite of and beyond its aggressive components. [p.103]

The Etiology of Dependency Problems: Childhood Issues

As we have noted in earlier chapters, researchers tell us that children suffering from both emotion and real separation from parents first protest angrily, then cry in despair, and finally become emotionally detached (Bowlby 1969, 1973, 1980). When mother or father returns, they behave indifferently; they do not risk a return to closeness (Fine 1988, Offit 1995).

The detached, affectless disposition of the cardiac personality to which we have referred frequently throughout this text emanates from a childhood where a warm attachment to a parent is either unavailable or inconsistent. To protect oneself, the cardiac personality learns in childhood to say, "Don't do me any favors! I don't need you!"

> Milton, an unemployed 56-year-old man, was referred to a low cost mental health clinic after he had a mild heart attack. When the social worker at intake told Milton that he would not have to pay a fee until he had a better income, Milton responded, "I don't need any favors. I don't want your help. I've learned to depend on no one."

> When the social worker tried to investigate with Milton why he was so reluctant to be given to, Milton responded, "I learned at an early age not to expect any handouts. Both my parents were alcoholics, they took care of their cravings and ignored mine. So, I learned to take care of myself starting at age one or maybe even before that."

Although there are not any statistical studies to suggest that cardiac personalities have suffered more than others from the premature death of one parent and have been alone as a child with the survivor, in my own practice and in those of my colleagues we have worked with many cardiac personalities where this has been the case. What we have noted in these situations is that as a child the patient was not only angry at one parent for dying but was furious at the surviving parent for demanding too much. In response to the deprivation and consequent burdens, the patient learned in childhood that it was safer to be socially isolated than to reach out and try to be attached.

> Nicole, a 42-year-old woman, was in treatment because she was "lonely and unmarried" and had some minor cardiac problems. Investigating her life, the therapist and Nicole

were able to determine that since her father died when she was 6 years old, Nicole had felt very depressed and was socially isolated.

In her fourth month of treatment, Nicole, able to cry for the first time in many years, said, "All my life I've missed a father. I feel so terribly gypped. I think there's a part of me that pushes men away, the way my father pushed me away. But, there's something else that's always bothered me. My mother was never a mother. Sometimes I think I've been her husband. At other times, she's been like a daughter to me. I've never had a normal life ever since my father died and my mother hasn't been of much help."

Another common problem I have noted among cardiac personalities, which also needs some statistical research, is that many of them either had or continue to have asthma. Although the idea that a person wheezing during an asthma attack signifies that he or she is crying out desperately for love is a controversial one (Sheridan and Kline 1984), there seems to be a strong similarity between an asthma attack and a heart attack. In both situations the individual is in a lot of pain and needs something akin to maternal support. In both crises the person is often out of touch with feelings and the body is used to discharge emotions. It may be conjectured that a loved child or adult breathes well and tends to be lighthearted. Perhaps an unloved child turns out to be cold-hearted and can't breathe too freely?

Over forty years ago, I treated a 20-year-old man whom we'll call Ogden. He had a chronic case of asthma. One of the most dramatic moments of therapy was when I agreed to begin treatment with him, the asthma abruptly stopped.

However, three months into therapy, when I told him I was going on vacation, he had an attack which bothered him throughout my week's vacation. On my return, the asthma went away. The same phenomenon occurred at spring and summer time: when I spoke about a separation, he had an attack; when I returned from vacation, the symptoms dramatically ceased.

During the course of the therapy Ogden and I discussed his childhood a great deal. He remembered a mother "who was there and not there." Said Ogden, "She was the kind of mother who could be loving and attentive one minute and not available another minute. At times I wanted to yell and scream at her. Maybe my asthma was a way to yell and scream?"

Alexander Lowen (1988) reported two cases of men who had asthma and then died prematurely of heart attacks. In the case of Jim, a 53-year-old man who had his first asthma attack at 6 months of age, Lowen reported that "Jim had been nursed for six months and then weaned which had constituted for him an overwhelming loss of his mother.... After he had cried his heart out to no avail, he had sucked in air and held his breath to stop the crying in the interest of survival" (p. 56). Jim continued to try to be very self-sufficient throughout his life. His mother's "failure to provide the support and nurturing he needed forced him to hold himself up by his will, which he continued to do throughout adulthood. To let down would have brought up the feeling of abandonment that, it seemed, he had so valiantly overcome as a child" (p. 57). When Jim was 55 years old, he suffered a fatal heart attack following the death of a sister to whom he was deeply attached.

In the second case, Lowen describes a man in his late forties who had a severe asthmatic condition. The man, whom we'll call Jack, recognized the importance of emotional factors in his illness and was hopeful that psychotherapy might ameliorate his condition. The breathing exercises he did during his consultation seemed to make him feel much better. However, because of a pending vacation, that is, a separation, the beginning of his therapy had to be postponed for a month. Jack never kept his appointment. His wife called to say he suffered a fatal heart attack.

I have often conjectured that wheezing is a substitute for crying and that many asthmatic children have held back their tears, feeling that it would only aggravate their interpersonal problems. As many writers have suggested (for example, Cortis 1995, Cousins 1983, English and Pearson 1945, Lowen 1988), the importance of crying to release tension and relieve heartache cannot be overstated. If the cardiac personality is helped as an adult to cry—something overlooked when he or she was a child—heart disease is afforded an opportunity to be reversed.

It would appear quite possible that the panic of adults who are having a heart attack is a similar type of panic that they experienced as children in response to heartbreak. Just as they did in childhood, they react to the threat their feelings pose by holding their breath and immobilizing their body on its deepest level, namely, the heart (Lowen 1988).

According to Norman Cousins (1983), one way to prevent heart attacks is to prevent panics. He states, "Panic intensifies underlying health problems. Panic can contract the blood vessels, disrupt normal heart rhythms, and even cause myocardial infarction" (p. 134). Thus, helping the person who had cardiac problems to master the panicky situations which emanate from childhood would seem to be an important factor in reversing heart disease.

Dependency in the Treatment Situation

Transference Issues

Perhaps one of the most difficult dimensions of working with cardiac personalities in psychotherapy is trying to resolve with them their complicated transference reactions which involve their dependency conflicts.

There are many reasons to account for the reluctance of cardiac personalities to form a sustained therapeutic alliance with the therapist. First and foremost, because cardiac personalities have learned to be mistrustful of any close interpersonal relationship, relating to the therapist on a sustained basis is not going to be an exception. Secondly, cardiac personalities have usually related to a host of doctors prior to meeting the therapist. Most of them have had no training in sensitizing themselves to the omnipotent and hostile defenses of cardiac patients and most of them are oblivious to their patients' dependency problems. Consequently, when cardiac personalities meet a psychotherapist, they are very inclined to say to themselves, "Another doctor! Who needs another doctor who won't care for me properly?" Thirdly, when and if the cardiac personality is able to expose dependency problems in the therapy, their expression is frequently intense and chaotic.

Let us look at some of the above-mentioned issues as they emerge in the clinical situation.

In previous chapters we have examined how difficult it is

for cardiac personalities to initiate a therapeutic relationship. Terrified of their dependency wishes, fearful that they will be placed in a vulnerable and powerless position, cardiac personalities frequently have to demean the therapist's expertise and authority. These issues become compounded in this day and age because the kind of treatment that most cardiac personalities need, long-term care, is being repudiated by many.

Inasmuch as third party payments and managed care are proliferating, and because their advocates champion short-term treatment, many cardiac personalities receive reinforcement from them in their quest to defeat the therapist's prescription of long-term care. If the therapist tries to refute the patient's argument, treatment, as we have seen, may be jeopardized.

Particularly at the beginning of treatment, but throughout its course, the therapist should bear in mind that depending on the therapist is always potentially threatening to the cardiac personality. Almost always the patient has a wish to move away from the therapist. The wish must be carefully listened to and respected and never opposed directly. With an accepting, nonthreatening attitude from the therapist, the cardiac patient may do what he or she usually really needs to do, remain in long-term treatment.

> Malcolm, a lonely 55-year-old bachelor, initially questioned being in psychotherapy. Although his cardiologist had strongly recommended it, Malcolm felt that the idea of sharing "troubles" with another person was "humiliating and not worthwhile." When his male therapist listened attentively and did not argue with him, Malcolm talked about his "always needing to control relationships," and resenting

"other people prying into my business."

Inasmuch as the therapist's attitude was very benign and nonconfrontational, Malcolm could explore his "depressing childhood" and see for himself how much he had to defend himself against passive yearnings and close interpersonal contacts.

The longer Malcolm was in therapy, the more he grew to like his therapist and the more he could see therapy as enhancing his life. He began to date women more, his interest in current events increased, and he became "more of a person." When the therapist showed how pleased he was with Malcolm's progress, Malcolm at first showed a similar pleasure. However, a few weeks later Malcolm decided that he had "enough of therapy" and wanted to quit at the end of the month. Realizing that his expression of pleasure must have disturbed Malcolm, the therapist stated, "As you know, it's always your decision when this therapy ends. But, tell me, how did you feel when I expressed a lot of pleasure about your therapeutic progress?" At first Malcolm said he felt "okay," but after a few silent moments of introspection, he became very angry.

"Goddamn it," Malcolm bellowed, "I hate the way I have to depend on you. I'm like a kid and you are my daddy. I resent your power and if I leave, I'll feel stronger." Tempted to argue with Malcolm, the therapist monitored his wish and said, "I can see how you'd feel much more comfortable without me in your life, but I will miss you if you go." After reflecting on the therapist's comments for a moment, Malcolm began to weep. He realized that his "warm attachment" to the therapist was "bothering" him. Yet, he felt he wanted to understand it better and decided to stay in therapy.

Although Malcolm decided to remain in treatment, many cardiac patients, despite the clinician's best efforts and most sensitive and tactful interventions, do leave the treatment. It is important at these times for the therapist to monitor his or her feelings of rejection and narcissistic injury and leave the door open for a possible return to therapy in the future. Many cardiac personalities, if they do not feel too dominated by the therapist, can leave therapy in the middle of it and then return at a later date.

> Louise, 61 years old, was a member of a support group of cardiac patients. After participating actively in the group for over 7 months, Louise felt that she wanted to try it on her own. Although the group leader and several of the members of the group realized that Louise was frightened to develop closer attachments with them, and shared their sentiments about this with Louise, she responded many times by saying, "I have to go."

> As the time drew near to Louise's departure, the leader and group members sadly accepted her decision. They shared their wish that someday soon Louise would return to the group. Feeling understood by the group and the leader, Louise was able "to take a sabbatical" of three months, felt "an empty space" while not attending the group, and returned.

Despite cardiac personalities strongly defending themselves against feeling and expressing their dependency feelings in the transference, when they do, their attachment to the therapist can become strong and their yearning can become great.

Kermit, a man in his mid-forties, was in treatment with a woman therapist for several reasons. He had a very tempestuous relationship with his wife, argued with his children constantly, was quite unsuccessful as an insurance agent, and he had a host of neurotic symptoms such as obsessions, compulsions, and phobias.

After fighting being a patient for over a year, during which time Kermit was very critical of the therapist's clothes, demeanor, office, and therapeutic techniques, Kermit changed his manner and tone quite dramatically. He told the therapist that anybody who could listen to his "hostile sermons" for so long and never retaliate is "quite a person."

Kermit's admiring and laudatory remarks became quite consistent and he began to fill every session with proclamations of his love toward the therapist. This moved to his having explicit desires to have meals with the therapist, go to the movies with her, and "have a friendship rather than a professional relationship."

Because the therapist was very sensitive to the fact that Kermit's extremely idealizing transference emanated from his strong, but disguised, wish to be her little boy, she was able to relate to him objectively but compassionately.

The therapist told Kermit that as she thought about him and their work together, she was having the impression that he would like to live with her and be taken care of by her. Flushing, stammering, and acutely embarrassed, Kermit tried to deny the truth of the therapist's interpretation. However, when the therapist told Kermit that all of his life he's been fighting closeness and was now fighting it with her, Kermit felt supported. Slowly he was able to bring out into the open his many fantasies to be a little boy, play with the therapist, eat with her, sleep with her, and go on vacation with her.

As the therapist patiently listened to Kermit's fantasies without much comment, Kermit could slowly arrange to make his marriage and other relationships more pleasureful and more mutually dependent. He became much warmer toward family members, business associates, and friends. Kermit stated to his therapist after 2 years of therapy, "I was so scared to love you, but you've made it easy. Now it's much easier to love others."

Resistances to Dependency

One of the common defenses of cardiac personalities is denial. As we have observed, they find it very difficult to acknowledge the truth about their omnipotent fantasies, hostile feelings, and dependent yearnings. When they enter therapy, denial is used frequently. They often claim they are immune from feelings of vulnerability, inferiority, envy, and particularly, dependency.

The resistances of cardiac personalities to depending on the therapy and the therapist are many and frequent. We have already noted their frequent claims that they do not need treatment. When they do agree to participate, they often come late for interviews, absent themselves from many, and constantly threaten to quit altogether. More subtle resistances are obsessing about the past, overemphasizing reality, or becoming excessively preoccupied with diet, exercise, meditation, and other features of cardiac rehabilitation which, though crucial, are only peripheral to their psychotherapy.

As we have stressed, it is always helpful to respect a patient's resistances, particularly at the beginning of treatment. This notion is especially pertinent to cardiac personalities, who constantly need to protect themselves from self-revelation.

My colleagues and I have noted that many of the cardiac patients who are in rehabilitation programs like to spend their psychotherapy sessions discussing their vegetarian fat-free diets, their exercise programs, and their medications. At first blush, we saw this as a resistance of the patient's which we tried to resolve quickly. In hindsight we realized we were too quick! What slowly dawned on us was that when cardiac patients talk about their food, exercise, and medication, they are unconsciously bringing their bodies to the therapist's attention. Symbolically, they are behaving like little children with a parent and asking the mother or father to gratify their dependent wishes. Although this is unconscious and indirect, it is a means of procuring dependency gratification when most other outlets are taboo.

When given free reign to discuss their diet, pills, and exercise, most cardiac patients eventually feel more relaxed with the therapist. They begin to sound like pleased children and then can move into conflict-ridden material more freely and with fewer disguises.

> Jeremiah, a single man in his early fifties, was in a therapy group for cardiac patients. Quiet at first, Jeremiah began to participate by describing how many of his aches and pains were lessening as he became very disciplined about exercising. Although the therapist and group members were somewhat bored listening to the details of Jeremiah's activities on the treadmill and bicycle, they correctly assumed that it was better for Jeremiah to talk about his exercise than not talk at all. Therefore, they asked him questions about his activities which reinforced his efforts to talk.

Eventually Jeremiah felt secure enough to share his lonely feelings with the group and he received sufficient help to begin dating women.

When cardiac personalities do get involved with the therapy, like everything else in their lives, they want quick results. Many times a cardiac patient, after only a few therapy sessions, will say that his or her marriage, job situation, or psychosomatic symptoms have not appreciably changed. The implication in these statements is that the therapist is not doing his job well and should be doing more.

Though it is tempting to point out reality to a patient who wants quick results after three or four sessions of therapy and tell the patient that good therapy takes time, it is rarely a helpful intervention. When cardiac patients are demanding quick results, a great deal is going on which is not too apparent. First, the patient is allowing himself or herself to be dependent and is demanding, "Why haven't you done something more for me lately?" Second, the patient's demands are so provocative that it can be inferred that the patient is unconsciously arranging to have a battle with the therapist. Finally, the patient is distorting the therapeutic process, not wishing to view it as a mutual effort.

In order to assist the patient to adapt to the therapeutic situation with a feeling of increasing safety, it is helpful, particularly at the beginning of treatment, to take the patient's complaints very seriously. One way for the clinician to convey that he or she is considering the patient's criticisms and demands with care is to ask questions about the patient's dissatisfactions.

Irma, age 46, was in treatment because she was very dissatisfied with her job as a computer specialist. She found her work dull and boring and was seriously considering changing professions. In her intake interview she mentioned that she had been divorced twice and wanted to find "a good man," but had been unsuccessful in her 3-month search.

After her first three interviews, her male therapist was aware of the fact that Irma was a very demanding woman who became easily dissatisfied with people and situations in a very short period of time. Consequently, he was well prepared when Irma, in her fourth session, asked him, "Do you feel we are getting anywhere?" Sensing her impatience but wanting to help her talk about her dissatisfactions, the therapist asked, "Do you?" Irma responded somewhat angrily and said, "I've already spent quite a bit of money and I'm still without a job I like and without a good man." The therapist acknowledged that the therapy and he had been very disappointing so far and was also making her irritable. Irma then went on to say that she wasn't getting her "money's worth" and "something had to change."

When the therapist asked what Irma would like changed, Irma again responded with irritation and said, "How am I supposed to know! You are the doctor." When the therapist asked Irma what she thought of what they had talked about so far, Irma answered, "You ask too many personal questions. You should give me advice."

When the therapist asked, "What area of your life would you like me to give advice about?" Irma answered, "I'd like to know what to say to men that will help me keep them. I'm always getting dumped. Inasmuch as you are a man, maybe you know what men want to hear." Here the therapist said, "Yes I am a man and right now we're not hitting it off too well. Perhaps you could tell me what bothers you about the questions I've been asking you that makes them 'too personal.'" Irma responded, "I guess I'm reluctant to get close to any man. I had a father who was very critical and I think I want to get back at him."

Slowly Irma began to understand how angry she was with men. She realized she was critical toward them in the same way her father was toward her. Her anger at men became the focus of the therapeutic work for many sessions and with this, her challenging the therapist diminished tremendously. She began to feel safer in forming a mutually dependent relationship with the therapist because he presented himself as less of a threat to her and more of an ally.

Although most cardiac personalities resist for long periods of time being dependent on their therapists, when they do permit their dependent wishes to emerge they can make psychotherapy a major preoccupation. They want to refer their friends and family members for therapy. They discuss psychotherapy wherever they go and with anybody who will listen. Their therapy, in effect, becomes a religion for them and they are eager to get anybody they can to convert to it.

What is often overlooked when patients become psychotherapy fanatics and try to make the clinician a guru is that the patients are really ambivalent about treatment. By trying to convince others that "It's the thing to do," they are really trying to diminish their own doubts. That is why they need people to reinforce the part of themselves which wants to remain in therapy.

In working with this resistance, it is important for the therapist to keep in mind that the psychotherapy fanatic has negative views about treatment and that eventually these views need to be expressed openly. Otherwise they can be acted out and the patient can prematurely leave treatment.

However, it is important for the therapist also to bear in mind that a patient who is consciously worshipping the therapy and the therapist needs a great deal of preparation before being confronted with negative feelings toward psychotherapy.

> Harold, a man in his mid-seventies, after overtly questioning the therapy and therapist for two months, became a "convert." He realized that looking at his feelings, fantasies, dreams, and history was "a very worthwhile avocation" and he was "slowly getting more and more people into the fold."

> His female therapist was very pleased initially when she noted Harold's dramatic shift in his attitude toward treatment. However, his obsessive preoccupation with therapy, his constant proselytizing, made her feel that the gentleman "doth protest too much." Yet, she knew it would take quite a bit of time before she could confront him with the meaning of his behavior.

> As Harold talked about "people who question therapy and need to be convinced," the therapist realized that Harold was projecting his own questions about treatment onto others. As the therapist asked Harold to shed some light for her on the resistances of "people who question therapy," Harold talked about their "latent distrust," "hostility," and "fear of emotions." The therapist made sure to be very accepting of the "people who question therapy" and, as Harold observed this, he became less critical of them. Slowly he could empathize and identify with them. Although it took several months before he could do so, Harold was eventually able to acknowledge some of his own doubts about treatment and examine their roots.

Countertransference Responses to Dependency Problems

An axiom of psychotherapeutic practice is that whatever therapists have not resolved in their own lives, they will not be able to help their patients resolve. Inasmuch as no therapist is a perfect psychological specimen, countertransference is ubiquitous. No therapist is exempt from problems with omnipotence, hostility, or dependency. We therapists would be well advised to accept our psychological problems as a given because we are just as human as our patients.

In his book *A Curious Calling: Unconscious Motivations for Practicing Psychotherapy*, Michael Sussman (1992) has clearly demonstrated that the marriages, work lives, and daily interactions of psychotherapists are as neurotic as most of their patients.

It would appear that if therapists want to be of real help to their patients, their job is to accept the fact that the man or woman in front of them is, in many ways, themselves. So, the question is not, "Do I have conflicts around dependency?" The more helpful question we probably should be asking ourselves is, "What dependency problems of mine are being activated with this unique patient, at this time?"

Many therapists, like many cardiac personalities, have strong yearnings to be dependent but have to deny these wishes. Often, they prefer to ponder the dependency problems of their patients rather than face their own. However, when the patient ignores the therapist, finds little to say about his or her effectiveness, and particularly talks about how other professionals are helpful, the therapist's dependency problems often do assert themselves.

Gloria, age 64, was in treatment with a male therapist because of depression, marital problems, and many somatic disorders. In her therapy, she was quite preoccupied with her bodily complaints and went into detail about them. When the therapist attempted to get Gloria to talk about her feelings, relationships, or daily interactions, Gloria frustrated him.

As the therapy moved on, Gloria made many references to physicians and others who were very helpful to her. At first, the therapist just listened, but after a while he found himself bristling because he was consistently shunned. But instead of examining what it meant to him to be ignored and what memories this activated for him, he made hostile interpretations. He told Gloria she was not facing her therapeutic responsibilities and was not dealing with her feelings and conflicts. Gloria, as she had all along, ignored the therapist's comments and quit therapy.

Being ignored is hardly ever a pleasant process. But it behooves therapists to know what uniquely gets stirred up for them when they are not the focus of their patient's attention. With more self-knowledge, they are better able to empathically deal with the patient's transference issues and resistances. If the therapist in the above case of Gloria had faced himself first, he might have been able to say to Gloria with some warmth, "You want to have little to do with me. Perhaps we can see what I'm doing that makes you want to stay away from me?" Maybe Gloria would have felt better understood and could have remained in treatment.

A countertransference problem which emerges frequently with cardiac personalities (and which was observed in the case of Gloria) is that the therapist becomes too eager to turn cardiac and other somatic problems into psychological problems.

Although the therapists always have their own theoretical predilections, values, and biases, imposing them on the patient often alienates the patient. Many cardiac patients need time before they are ready to face their personal problems.

> Forty-nine-year-old Frank was being seen in a community mental health center. Referred by a physician because of migraine headaches, gastrointestinal disturbances, insomnia, and depression, Frank spent a great deal of his time in sessions obsessing about his physical aches and pains. After a few months of listening to his "boring monologues," his female therapist became more active. She began to interpret to Frank that his bodily ills were a manifestation of his resentment and dependency. At first, Frank just ignored the therapist. When she persisted, Frank's bodily complaints became more intense and excessive and before too long he had to be hospitalized.

One of the lessons which we can derive from the case of Frank is that bodily symptoms serve defensive purposes. They protect the patient from facing unbearable ideas and feelings. Consequently, they must be understood and respected by the therapist. If confronted too soon in the treatment and without sufficient tact or empathy, the patient's condition can become exacerbated. Therefore, therapists, like patients, should learn to modulate their harsh judgments—the theme of our next chapter.

7

From Harsh
Judgments
to Constructive
Communication

One of the most obvious characteristics of cardiac personalities is their strong propensity to make harsh judgments of others as well as of themselves. Driven by perfectionistic standards, bombarded by hostile fantasies, unable to tolerate childish yearnings and human vulnerabilities in themselves and others, cardiac personalities are rarely able to accept family, friends, colleagues, and themselves as they are. Hence, the social isolation that seems to pervade their lives becomes quite understandable.

In order to better sensitize ourselves to how and why harsh and punitive standards are so much part of cardiac personalities' *modus vivendi*, we have to take another look at their early childhoods. Childhood is the time when we develop our standards for living and incorporate ethical and moral imperatives into our superego, the part of the mind that is the storehouse of parental and societal admonitions and ideals.

In his paper "On Narcissism," Sigmund Freud (1914)

speaks of an "ego ideal" which measures the individual's daily behavior. He points out that the ego ideal is "constantly watching" the person, approving or disapproving of behavior, much like most parents do with their children. Freud points out here that the ego ideal is formed by introjecting parental criticism and is reinforced by those who train and teach the child.

In his later papers (for example, "The Ego and the Id") Freud (1923) views the superego as having "a harsh voice" because it is utilized to prohibit the expression of hostile and other forbidden impulses. Freud and other dynamically oriented therapists who further developed the notion of the superego (for example, English and Pearson 1945, Glover 1960) have shown that the more hatred there is in the child's heart, the more he or she will have to repudiate this hatred by developing a harsh superego.

How and why does the child repudiate hostile wishes and then form a harsh and punitive superego? It will be recalled that when youngsters feel emotionally neglected and/or abandoned, their initial reactions are usually protest and hostility (Bowlby 1969, 1973, 1980). However, most children cannot feel free to discharge their angry feelings because they anticipate retaliation and/or loss of love. Consequently, they repress their hostility and instead become desperate and withdrawn.

Inasmuch as "would-be cardiac personalities" usually experience their parents as sadistic and brutal, rather than oppose them, they introject their parents' punitive voices into their consciences or superego. The more hatred they feel, the more retaliation they expect and the more they become subject to a punitive, harsh superego.

The psychoanalyst Edward Glover (1960), in discussing

the evolution of the superego, states:

> The child, projecting his hostile fantasies onto the imagos of the parents, creates imagos that are more powerful and draconic in morality than the parents actually are.... As he continues to introject parental imagos, the child introjects these distorted elements also, with the result that his unconscious conscience can be more severe (sadistic)...than are the realistic inferences of the parents. [p.142]

Glover's notion that because the child is so frightened of his or her hostility and the retaliation that it might provoke forms a punitive superego, more punitive than the parents' realistic admonitions, has important implications for understanding and treating the cardiac personality. As a child, the cardiac personality could not feel safe in sharing angry thoughts with and toward parental figures. To make sure of preserving parental love, cardiac personalities as children became harsh parents to themselves. Early in life, they admonished themselves, often spanking themselves and saying, "Bad boy!" "Bad girl!"

As we listen to the childhoods of cardiac personalities in psychotherapy, we hear about children who lacked what Schafer (1983) has called "the loving and beloved superego." Rather, these children had sadistic superegos that constantly condemned them. They felt overpowered as they heard the internalized voices of aggressively demanding parents. Frightened of rebelling against these voices, they submitted to them. And, if they were inclined to feel or act on their aggression, they used their harsh superegos to tell themselves "to be seen and not heard."

As these children with "unloving superegos" continued to interact with others, they had a tendency to admonish others in the way they were disciplined. They severely reprimanded dolls and animals and then moved on to do the same with siblings and peers. By the time they were in their teens, the children we are describing "blossomed" into cardiac personalities. Frightened of their anger, they repressed it and became very vigilant about "right and wrong" regarding themselves and others. Still yearning to be loved, they were very perfectionistic, hoping their omnipotent strivings would impress their parents. Frustrated by the lack of parental response, they became very agitated, hid their dependency yearnings, and felt more and more stress. Their stress, as we know, became converted into somatic disorders like heart disease.

In this chapter, we want to observe how the cardiac personality's harsh judgment affects marital and other love relationships, work interactions, and daily life. We also want to discuss how their harsh superego can be tamed in the treatment situation.

Harshness in Marriage

One of the common and serious problems of cardiac personalities, particularly in marriage and love relationships, is their strong tendency to project their own punitive superegos onto their partners. Once the partner is cast as a punitive disciplinarian, cardiac personalities feel controlled and dominated by the partner and have strong wishes to rebel against him or her.

Although there is usually some reality in the way cardiac personalities experience their punitive partners, that is, the partners may be realistically critical and punitive, what is important for the helping professional to keep in mind is that cardiac personalities frequently want, albeit unconsciously, to be married to a punitive spouse. Rather than confront a self image that is one of an angry, guilt-ridden child who deserves consistent punishment, cardiac personalities arrange for their spouses to be held accountable for their misery. According to many cardiac personalities, the spouse is the one who is angry and unloving, and therefore should be hated. Cardiac personalities are often convinced that they would be much happier if they had a more loving spouse and often try to prove that.

Husbands and wives who have extramarital affairs and/or move to other partners to avoid being punished (Strean 1995a) inevitably come face to face with their own self-hatred and don't usually find another partner to be of much assistance. Unless they are helped through psychotherapy or group support to see that they are busily punishing themselves, their misery in love relationships tends to continue.

> Ed, a 41-year-old man, came to psychotherapy because he was "in a miserable marriage." He described his wife as "putting a noose" around his neck and "dominating the hell" out of him. Ed was sexually impotent with his wife most of the time but blamed his sexual difficulties on her. "She acts like a mother with me and makes me feel like a little boy," bellowed Ed in anger.

> To buttress his conviction that he was "a victim of circumstances," Ed became involved in an extramarital affair and was able to boast about how potent he was with his paramour. "I know I'm a man because I'm always very sexual with my girlfriend. If my wife acted the way my girlfriend does, I'd have a happy marriage," said Ed with much

assurance to his male therapist.

Over time Ed was able to see that his sexual problems were largely of his own making. Of enormous help to him was going away with his girlfriend for a week where living with her on a daily basis made her seem as if she were his wife. Seeing her as a wife, he became sexually impotent with his girlfriend.

After close to a year of twice a week psychotherapy, Ed was able to say to his therapist, "When I live with a woman, I start to feel that she's big and I'm small. She starts to become a mother and even smells like my own mother. Maybe she doesn't want to control me as much as I think she does, but I'm a goner as soon as I feel she's more than a date."

Although making the partner a superego is a frequent happenstance among cardiac personalities, many cardiac personalities arrange to be a punitive superego with their partners. Rather than demean themselves for their own imperfections, vulnerabilities, and forbidden wishes, they criticize their partners for being human. And, instead of masochistically submitting to their spouses or partners, they become the sadist and arrange for their partner to suffer. In effect they relate to the partner the way their parents punitively related to them.

Dolores, 45 years old, was in therapy because she found herself "constantly resenting" her husband. Although she mentioned in her intake interview that her criticisms could be "very intense," in her therapy sessions with her female therapist she spent almost all of her time reporting how her husband "acted like an ass." Because her therapist remained neutral as she listened to Dolores' complaints, Dolores was able to get in touch with the harsh voices of her own super-ego. Eventually she realized that she sounded like her mother yelling at her father. After a few months of therapy she could insightfully state to her therapist, "It's easier to beat up my husband than to beat up myself. It's a good thing he wants me to be his evil conscience."

While cardiac personalities tend to form subgroups either making the partner the punitive superego or becoming one themselves, many cardiac personalities take turns with their partners. In some ways it is like a sadomasochistic relationship wherein the partners are dynamically similar and unconsciously alternate as to whom is going to be the boss.

Charles and Bessie were a couple in their sixties. Both suffered from cardiac problems and both acknowledged that throughout their 35-year-old marriage there was hardly a day that was free from altercations.

Charles and Bessie both came from broken homes and both witnessed a great deal of friction between their parents.

In their day-to-day interactions, they found many ways to demean the other. Charles was berated by Bessie daily for being mechanically inept, and Bessie was constantly criticized by Charles for her insufficient attention to the appearance of the house. Each had certain specified areas to criticize and be criticized in. Unconsciously they both "enjoyed" being a harsh taskmaster as well as a victim of a harsh taskmaster. It was not until they had heart problems that they considered getting some help for their severe marital problems.

Charles and Bessie were at the same level of emotional maturity and both had severe superego problems. As is true in all marital difficulties, there are no sinners and no saints. Both partners tend to contribute their fair share to the conflicts!

Harsh Judgments at Work

That bosses can be experienced as punitive superegos by their workers is well-known. Many cardiac personalities are and have been task masters who enjoy dominating and reprimanding their subordinates. What has not been given much consideration is how those in authority can behave in such a way that those under them become punitive superegos for them. Many teachers can act in a provocative, passive-aggressive manner so that their students mobilize and constantly overtly or covertly criticize their attitudes and behavior. The same dynamic has been observed with executives, administrators, and politicians with their subordinates.

What seems to transpire in these situations is that those in command often experience their own superior positions as ones they don't deserve. It is as if these individuals feel they have stolen the top job from a parental figure and, therefore, the job in their minds does not belong to them. In fantasy, they are the recipients of stolen goods and have to return what they have taken.

Adam was a 55-year-old man who was a chairman of an English department in a major university. Everyone in Adam's department and many others throughout the university supported the idea that he become chairman of the department because of his excellent capabilities as a teacher and researcher.

After just a few months of being chairman, Adam managed to antagonize most of the faculty and many of the students in his English department. They resented his unilateral decision-making, his long-winded monologues, and his emotional unavailability.

By the time Adam sought psychotherapy, he was suffering from many somatic difficulties including heart problems. In addition, he had uncontrollable temper tantrums, insomnia, and depression.

When Adam and his male therapist attempted to investigate what Adam did to contribute to his difficulties with his colleagues, they learned a great deal by examining one of Adam's administrative practices. Almost daily Adam was meeting with faculty members, students, or both to learn from them what he had been doing to weaken the morale of the department. As the dynamics of some of these meetings were explored in the therapy, it became quite clear that Adam received considerable gratification from being reprimanded. He pointed out in therapy that he could feel "a certain relief" after being admonished. Although he initially rationalized his behavior with colleagues by referring to it as "democratic leadership," Adam discovered other meanings of his behavior. Slowly he learned that he "felt a strong obligation to get [his] wrists slapped."

As Adam carefully and comprehensively investigated with his therapist his wish for punishment from his colleagues, he learned that he had secretly gratified a fantasy of "beating them up" when he became chairman. Stated Adam with much conviction, "I felt that I knocked out everybody in the department and grabbed the job they all wanted. Now I have to be knocked out."

In effect, Adam made his colleagues a punitive superego so that he could be punished for his imagined sins. Feeling like an oedipal victor, Adam had to make all of his subordinates into father figures who would destroy him.

Many of the problems of the workaholic that we have alluded to in previous chapters are also superego problems. Feeling guilty about achievements and the pleasure that can be derived from them, many workaholics work overtime as a form of punishing themselves. The workplace becomes like a tyrannical parent and the workaholic must submit to all kinds of pressures from the parent.

A fairly common problem in the workplace and one that plagues many cardiac personalities is competition with colleagues. Although in many ways a recapitulation of old sibling problems, when colleagues "tattle tale" on each other to the boss and others, superego issues are also operative. The gossiper or tattler is, in effect, demeaning others for what are superego problems of his or her own. If individuals have wishes to be late for work or to shirk chores, but feel guilty about these desires, they can derive gratification by talking about colleagues who are guilty of these "crimes." Gossipers may also derive some delight seeing someone other than themselves being punished for what they would like to do.

Beverly, a 45-year-old lawyer, spent a lot of her time in her law firm "telling" on colleagues. She made a daily habit out of telling her boss which colleagues were not arriving on time, weren't putting in enough time on assignments, or "faked being sick" to stay out of work.

When Beverly's activities alienated her from her peers, so much so that several of them stopped talking to her, Beverly became depressed, lost a lot of weight, and seemed suicidal.

Beverly was eventually able to acknowledge that she was very envious of her colleagues who didn't take their work as seriously as she did. She would have liked to have been in their shoes, but was too inhibited and too guilty to try. Instead she attempted to inhibit colleagues from being rebellious, something she secretly wanted to be but could not face in herself.

It took Beverly close to 2 years before she could resolve her superego conflict.

Many work problems are superego problems. In order to resolve them, individuals who suffer from them must face the punitive voices within themselves and discover why they need to hold on to these voices.

Harsh Judgments in Daily Life

One of the consequences of having a harsh punitive superego is that it is almost always active, regardless of the situation that the individual is in. In addition, if a man or woman starts to feel less burdened in marriage, the punitive voices can become louder and more frequent at work. And, if they do not appear in marriage or work, they emerge in daily life.

Individuals with powerful superegos feel like convicts who have escaped from jail and are constantly awaiting being caught. If the phone rings, they worry about who is going to incriminate them. If the boss greets them, they wonder when they are going to be fired. If they see a policeman, they wonder when they are going to be arrested. Never exempt from guilt, they are forever arranging for punishment.

What has not received sufficient attention by those of us who work with cardiac personalities is how their punitive superegos are a major factor in their stress. Yet, inasmuch as they are always wondering when they are going to be divorced, fired, arrested, or berated, life can rarely be pleasureful for them. Many cardiac personalities, when they begin to enjoy themselves, become very anxious. They are sure that the axe is going to fall any minute because they have not submitted to their tyrannical parents, who appear in the form of a spouse or boss.

In daily life the punitive superego becomes a constant threat that can always increase the individual's heartbeat. For example, a woman driving to work may be worried that she should be punished for leaving her home with the bed unmade and dishes unwashed. Upset that she is not being sufficiently responsible, she tells herself that if she gets home from work earlier than usual she can take care of her domestic chores. She tries to get to work faster so that she can get home earlier, but while accelerating her car, she worries about being arrested for speeding. Very agitated by the time she gets to work and feeling very irritable, she worries that her colleagues will not find her acceptable. This puts further pressure on her. Eventually she becomes both breathless and light-headed; her punitive superego has put her in enormous stress.

The reason it is important to understand how the punitive superego is a major cause of stress is because many individuals, including mental health professionals, think that if a person modifies a stressful situation or leaves it, the stress will disappear. If a punitive superego is present in the psyche, environmental manipulation rarely produces significant constructive change.

> Calvin, age 64, was in psychotherapy after he had been diagnosed as having severe heart disease. One of Calvin's issues was his constantly moving his residence to another town or within the same city. In a period of 5 years, he had moved his home six times.
>
> As Calvin and his female therapist took a look at his life, it became quite clear that Calvin was very paranoid. He was constantly convinced that neighbors and others resented him and were "after" him. Rather than face his strong hostility and fear of retaliation, he blamed his problems on his current external environment. It seemed quite logical to him that if his stress was caused by his neighborhood, he should move. He did not recognize that he was projecting his punitive superego onto his neighbors.

Another superego problem that cardiac personalities frequently manifest is "injustice collecting" (Bergler 1969). Whether they are concerned with politics, sports, friends, or family, they are constantly preoccupied with issues like inequality and unfairness. They manage always to see how they or someone else is being exploited. Of course, the improprieties that preoccupy them get them indignant. Consequently, they always are under a great deal of stress.

The reason injustice collectors suffer as much as they do is because they project their harsh superegos onto those they accuse of being unfair and then fight them overtly and/or in fantasy. What is not clear to injustice collectors is that the fights they are involved in are never-ending. Inasmuch as the fights are internal ones—they are battling the voices of their own punitive and harsh superego—they do not want to win. To repudiate the voices of their conscience would be experienced as destroying mother, father, or other figures of authority with whom they have identified.

Very often injustice collectors are champions of social causes where they constantly identify with the underdog and oppose arbitrary authorities. Their indignation feels justified as they battle poverty, crime, or war. What is important for the helping professional to keep in mind is that injustice collectors are rarely eager to resolve injustices. Rather, they want to continue battling the parental figures on whom they have projected their harsh consciences.

> Dorothy, age 40, was an attorney for the Legal Aid Society. She worked day and night for impoverished clients who were mistreated by government officials and others. At her first consultation with her male therapist, she told him that she was always in a rage and frequently had temper tantrums as she dealt with her adversaries.

> It took Dorothy close to a year of therapy before she could see that she was really in futile battles with her punitive father whose harsh voice she had internalized during her childhood.

> When Dorothy's therapy enabled her to separate her fight with her father from the realistic problems of clients, she could become much more effective in her legal work.

The Etiology of the Harsh Superego—Childhood Events

At the beginning of this chapter we alluded to some of the childhood conflicts of cardiac personalities who have been afflicted with a punitive superego. To enrich our understanding, it might be helpful to look at some of the actual childhood experiences of cardiac personalities who revealed very harsh superegos in their treatment.

One of the common childhood problems of cardiac personalities is that they were loved conditionally by their parents. Depending on what the parents valued, the child had to strive very hard to please them. If the parents did not have their own narcissistic wishes fulfilled by their sons or daughters, they stopped loving their children and often showed a lot of hatred toward them.

When children are subjected to conditional love, they are placed in an enormous dilemma. Because they resent being loved arbitrarily, they want to rebel. But, if they rebel, they will lose the very love they want. Sometimes they try to deny that they need parental approval and develop what Erikson (1950) has called *a negative identity*. They do the opposite of what their parents sanction and try to convince themselves and the world that they are unaffected by parental admonitions. This rarely works out successfully.

> Ethan, a 61-year-old man, had suffered from two heart attacks. When he began his psychotherapy, he attributed his cardiac problems to the fact that he never enjoyed his work as a dentist. He strongly believed that he should have been an English professor or a journalist.

> When Ethan's childhood was investigated in therapy, he described both of his parents as "very demanding and very authoritarian." Ethan also stressed that they had very definite attitudes about how he should conduct his life. One of their demands was that Ethan become a lawyer and go into politics. A second pressure was that he marry a woman from an affluent home.

As the parental demands escalated, Ethan began to rebel more and more. Instead of studying to be a lawyer, he became interested in the sciences and turned to dentistry. Rather than marrying a rich woman, he married one who was poverty-stricken.

Although Ethan derived some gratification from his negative identity, he realized in his therapy that in his work and love life he was not doing what gave him real pleasure but what would upset his parents. In addition, he felt quite guilty about defying his parents and that only compounded his misery.

Assuming a negative identity is, at best, only a temporary solution. It is a stab at the voices of the superego but rarely can be enjoyed on a sustained basis because of the guilt it induces.

In my own work with cardiac personalities I have observed a superego problem which only a few of my colleagues have also noted. How common it is is still difficult for me to assess. The issue to which I am referring is one where the child hears contradictory commands from his or her parents. Mother may want the child to be neat and clean while father directly or indirectly champions messiness. One parent may want the child to be active while the other extols passivity. Father may discuss sexual issues while mother avoids it completely.

When children are exposed to conflicting demands and values by their parents, they are placed in a very stressful situation. Eager to please both parents, they risk being admonished by one of them, regardless of what they do or feel. Consequently, they are constantly under tension because sooner or later the axe will fall.

What seems to occur internally with children who have been tormented by discordant voices of parents is that they develop a corrupt superego that is always ready to say, "You are doing something wrong!" These patients know no peace and life is usually quite miserable.

> Florence, a single 32-year-old woman, came for therapy because she was very depressed, occasionally suicidal, and "loathed" herself much of the time. She had numerous symptoms including phobias, compulsions, obsessions, and somatic disorders. Although she was a competent high school teacher, Florence was always questioning how effective she was with her students.
>
> After a year and a half of intensive therapy (three times a week) Florence realized that she was trying to placate the voices of two harsh parents who each demanded very different things from her. Her father, covertly and overtly, seemed to want Florence to be a boy. He pushed her to be very athletic, laughed with glee when she was belligerent, and ignored her when she was interested in traditional feminine activities such as cooking and sewing. In sharp contrast to her father, Florence's mother extolled passivity. When Florence was quiet or doing nothing, mother embraced her. However, whenever Florence was active, mother was very critical of her.
>
> Florence, eager to please both of her parents, could "never do anything right." She grew up to be her "own worst enemy." Unable ever to feel loved by both parents, she could never develop "a beloved superego." As a result stress was always part of her life.

Another etiological factor in the formation of a punitive superego is when a child lives with only one parent and the single parent makes the child an adult companion rather than a son or daughter. The child feels pressured to live an adult's life and resents it. Eager to break away but guilty for even contemplating it, the child develops a punitive superego that censures the child every time he or she thinks of being autonomous.

> George, a single, 52-year-old man, was in therapy for depression, somatic difficulties, and "extreme loneliness."
>
> Early in his treatment, George talked about the fact that his father died when he was 8 years old and his mother never remarried. Lamented George, "I had to be her husband and I could never feel good if I had my own life. I guess I never did have my own life."

The punitive superego in the cardiac personality is clearly one of the major contributors to the individual's stress and unhappiness. Almost always, the patient cannot overcome the difficulty unless he or she has some therapy.

Therapeutic Considerations in Reducing the Harsh Superego

One of the tasks in psychotherapy with cardiac personalities is to help them reduce the severity of their harsh superego. The main way to accomplish this task is by providing these patients with a therapist who is consistently experienced as a benign superego. In contrast to the patient's parental introjects, the therapist accepts the patient unconditionally and consistently empathizes with the patient's struggles, pains, and emotions. Eventually the patient identifies with the therapist's perspective and introjects a new superego that is less punitive and less harsh.

Providing the cardiac personality with "a corrective emotional experience" (Alexander and French 1946) not only comes from the therapist's "unconditional positive regard" (Rogers 1951) but through a careful analysis of the patient's transference reactions. As cardiac patients see how they distort the therapist and turn him or her into a harsh and inconsistent superego, they begin to see how they are constantly provoking and seeking punishment in their daily lives.

Transference Reactions

One of the most common transference reactions which most patients in psychotherapy manifest, and one which is particularly evident in the therapy of cardiac patients, is making the therapist a punitive superego. By projecting one's punitive superego onto the therapist, the patient not only seeks the punishment desired but also has the opportunity of opposing a seemingly tyrannical parent. If the therapist does not get manipulated by the patient's neurotic ploys, the latter may be able to diminish the severity of his or her punitive superego.

> Helen, a 46-year-old woman, came for treatment after her only child, a daughter, left home for college. Separating from her daughter activated many problems for Helen. She became severely depressed, lost interest in sex, argued incessantly with her husband, and quit her job as a librarian.

Although Helen initially responded very positively to her female therapist's empathetic and benign approach and became less depressed and more interested in her life, after a few months of therapy the symptoms returned. She became as depressed and miserable as she had been when she entered treatment.

When the therapist took note of Helen's negative therapeutic reaction and wondered what she was not doing for Helen, Helen had an interesting transference reaction. She told the therapist that the latter was "faking" an accepting attitude, and really hated Helen. Wishing to maintain her accepting attitude, the therapist asked Helen, "What do you think I could possibly hate you for?" Helen had a long list of complaints that she was sure the therapist was voicing behind Helen's back. She told the therapist, "You must hate me for not making progress in therapy, for being a little baby and being so dependent on my daughter, for not wanting sex with my husband, and more."

When the therapist stated, "You apparently don't feel I'm here to help you feel better and to understand yourself more but instead I want to berate you!" Helen began to sob. She pointed out that the therapist's description of her attitude toward Helen was an exact replica of her mother's attitude toward her.

Over time, Helen could see how she was consistently projecting her punitive superego onto the therapist and making her into a very harsh mother. By maintaining an unconditionally warm and empathetic attitude and consistently analyzing the transference, the therapist could help Helen like herself much more.

Another transference reaction of cardiac personalities

which also appears quite frequently is one in which the patient projects his or her forbidden impulses onto the therapist and then becomes the therapist's punitive superego. This arrangement permits the patient to discharge a great deal of aggression and vicariously consider his or her unacceptable wishes.

> Isaac was 60 years old when he was referred to his male therapist because of frequent arguments with his wife, relatives, and colleagues. His work as an accountant was in jeopardy because he had many altercations with his clients.
>
> In exploring the roots of Isaac's interpersonal problems, it became quite clear that Isaac had much difficulty feeling close to people. When the possibility arose, he handled his anxiety by arguing. When the therapist made an interpretation of this dimension of his life and said, "You seem to find intimacy uncomfortable and need to keep a distance from people," Isaac became angry with the therapist. He told him, "You want love too much and are a very dependent person who in many ways is too passive."
>
> Because the therapist never denied or affirmed Isaac's "diagnostic assessments" of him, Isaac could eventually begin to think of his own fears of loving and being loved and his own passivity. As he felt less guilt because he could identify with the therapist's nondefensiveness, he began to assert himself more constructively and make many less harsh judgments of others.

It usually takes awhile before the patient's transference reactions are explicit. When they are, they provide an excellent opportunity to help the patient master the toxic introjects which are in his or her psyche.

Resistances

Although a harsh superego causes considerable pain and inhibits pleasure, it is difficult to give up. It will be recalled that when children erect a punitive superego in their psyches, they often do this in order to censor sadistic and other forbidden wishes which have been long repressed.

One of the resistances which a cardiac personality with a harsh superego frequently manifests in treatment is that he or she becomes an arch-conformist. This patient arrives on time for every session, pays fees promptly, is most courteous to the therapist, listens to the therapist's comments very attentively, and tries hard to fulfill the therapist's wishes. Devoid of affect, this patient often behaves like an automaton in the therapeutic situation.

It is very difficult to help very conforming patients to resolve their resistances. They often are millions of miles away from realizing that their compliant behavior protects them from feeling and acting upon their murderous wishes. Rather, they strive hard to behave themselves without thinking too much about what they are doing. Just as they found it difficult in the past to be critical of their parents and other figures of authority, they rarely find fault with the therapist or the therapeutic process.

In working with the compliant patient, who often can become boring to the therapist, it is important for clinicians to remind themselves that the compliant behavior protects the patient against the danger of being bombarded by intense and overwhelming wishes to rebel. It is also helpful to these patients for the therapist not to be seduced by the patient's acquiescent behavior. A quiet and neutral attitude over a long period of time usually releases the patient's rebellious desires.

Janet, 52 years old, came for therapy because she had migraine headaches, chronic constipation, insomnia, and a host of other bodily complaints. A single woman, she was very unsuccessful in meeting men. When she did, she was not able to sustain relationships.

In her treatment with a male therapist, Janet was extremely polite, always conformed to the requests made of her, and often praised the therapist for his "brilliant" understanding. When the therapist maintained his neutral stance and did not overtly react to Janet's compliments and other ingratiating behavior, Janet slowly became irritated with him. At first her irritation came out in dreams where she found herself yelling at "male school teachers who never offered anything." Later, she began to voice her disapproval of male physicians and other helping professionals.

When the therapist had enough data accumulated, he said to Janet in her eighth month of treatment, "You are now much freer to be yourself. You can say how you honestly feel about men whom you resent. But, you are having difficulty telling me your complaints about me." At first, Janet denied having any resentment toward the therapist. However, when her migraine headaches and other somatic symptoms intensified, she could accept the therapist's comment that she would rather suffer than tell the therapist what she resented about him because she worried that her remarks would make him suffer.

Interventions like those described above eventually helped Janet get in touch with strong murderous wishes toward both of her parents. As she could speak about them, her symptoms diminished and her need for a powerful superego declined.

As observed with Janet, many cardiac personalities cope with their increased resentment toward therapy and the therapist by becoming sicker. Often they are unconsciously saying to the therapist, "What you are doing is making me feel worse. Maybe if I continue to suffer, you will respond to me in a loving way!"

Also, cardiac personalities frequently demonstrate what Freud (1923) termed *the negative therapeutic reaction*. It will be recalled that what Freud referred to here was the patient who verbalizes all the insights and interpretations which the therapist offers but never gets better. Freud attributed the patient's not making progress to his or her inability to enjoy pleasure because of a punishing superego. Modern therapists (for example, Fine 1982) believe that the patient who does not make progress, in addition to a punitive superego, is secretly trying to defeat the therapist. This patient, in many ways, wants the therapist to suffer but cannot say this directly.

Sometimes the clinician can observe increased somatization and the negative reaction in the same patient.

> Ken, a 47-year-old man, was referred to treatment by his physician, who felt Ken's obesity, asthma, backaches, and headaches had a strong psychological basis.
>
> In the first few months of therapy with a female clinician, Ken behaved in a submissive, compliant manner. When his therapist responded neutrally to this behavior, Ken became very masochistic in and out of treatment. His symptoms intensified, he became impotent with his wife, and he began to be very forgetful.
>
> The therapist interpreted Ken's exacerbation of problems as an expression of his disappointment with the therapy and the

therapist. Ken agreed with the therapist's observations. He even provided genetic and dynamic proof that he "always aimed to be Number One" and was "furious when this did not come about."

Despite Ken's insights his symptoms did not abate, but worsened. When the therapist felt defeated by Ken and acknowledged this openly, Ken's reaction was most illuminating. He asked the therapist if she was ready to throw Ken out of treatment. The therapist asked Ken, "Do you think that's a good idea?" Ken provided another revealing insight. He said, "Since I couldn't be number one and be the only guy in your life, I guess I've wanted to torture you. If you throw me out, I won't be able to torture you. I guess I'll have to get better."

Ken did get better when he could begin to talk more directly about his dependency yearnings and aggression. The more he could do this, his harsh superego diminished in intensity and he began to assert himself more constructively.

The case of Ken demonstrates once again the strong sadistic component in the psyche of the individual with a harsh superego. As we also noted in the above case, cardiac personalities with punitive consciences can induce strong countertransference reactions.

Countertransference Reactions

One of the reasons that patients with harsh superegos induce strong and frequent countertransference reactions is because their behavior is very deceptive and the therapist often doesn't know just what the patient is really feeling and trying to achieve. The patient's extremely cooperative behavior can mask hostility; his or her defiance can cover up dependency yearnings. Because the patients we are focusing on are very ambivalent about many issues, the therapist often doesn't know in what direction the patient wants to go at a given time.

One countertransference problem which emerges quite frequently when therapists become unsure about the patient's progress is to give advice to the patient. Anxious about the patient's lack of progress, overwhelmed by his or her constant uncertainty, and bored by the patient's affectless way of relating, by actively guiding the patient can the therapists temporarily dissipate their uncomfortable feelings. When the patient goes back and forth on a course of action for a long time, it is tempting to tell the patient which way to go.

The problem with advice giving is that it may offer a temporary respite to the therapist and to the patient as well, but it rarely resolves the superego and other problems which need to be addressed.

> Lila, age 56, was in treatment at a mental health clinic with a female social worker. She was being seen for many problems: a difficult marriage, an unsatisfying job, depression, sexual conflicts, phobias, and numerous somatic difficulties.

> In her treatment, Lila spoke in a monotone about her many hardships. She listened to the therapist's comments with interest but hardly ever related to them. Rather, she continued to sound very helpless as the therapist attempted to assist her in coping with her marital and work problems.

After 4 months of weekly treatment, when Lila showed no improvement, Ms. M., the therapist, began to give her advice. She told Lila to speak up on the job and at home and even suggested what she should say to her boss and her husband. However, after Lila listened attentively to Ms. M., she asked for further advice. She became extremely helpless in trying to act on Ms. M's advice and seemed to regress further and further.

Ms. M. finally became exasperated with Lila and transferred her to another therapist.

What we learn from the case of Lila is that patients who are indecisive and helpless can induce similar feelings in the therapist. Unless therapists can face their discomfort, they may be inclined to become overactive in the therapeutic situation. This only stimulates further helplessness and passivity in the patient, and therapeutic movement is usually impeded.

Because patients with superego problems can be very frustrating in the treatment situation, therapists need to constantly monitor their own anger. Sometimes the therapist's anger erupts but its expression only helps the therapist reduce tension for brief moments. It rarely is of any assistance to the patient.

Morris, 54 years old, was in therapy for a variety of problems. He had extreme difficulties coping with his aged parents, was constantly annoying his wife and children, was depressed, and was constantly on the verge of being fired from his job.

In his treatment with a male therapist, Morris had very little to say. When the therapist tried to stimulate him to talk,

Morris responded with one- or two-word answers. The therapist, Dr. P, became increasingly irritated with Morris' extreme passivity. After offering advice, many interpretations, and loads of questions, all of which yielded no emotional response, Dr. P. yelled at Morris and told him he was "rigid, passive-aggressive, stubborn, and provocative."

Initially Morris seemed to be unaffected by Dr. P.'s vituperative behavior, but after a couple of sessions he gave Dr. P. some sound advice. Said Morris, "I realize that talking is very difficult for me. But if a kid doesn't want to eat, should you stuff him with food? If an adult doesn't want to talk, it doesn't help to stuff him with words."

Morris also advised Dr. P. that though he didn't make any progress in therapy with him, he now knew what kind of therapist he needed.

Dealing with the harsh superego of the cardiac personality is a difficult task for both patient and therapist. However, if the therapist can withstand the frustration of the patient's affectlessness, indecisiveness, and obsessiveness, the patient eventually feels safe enough to release his aggression and other forbidden wishes. When forbidden desires are discussed openly and directly in the therapy, the patient usually begins to feel less oppressed by a harsh superego and more able to relate intimately and communicate constructively.

8

Love Is
the Answer

When omnipotent desires are diminished and hostility is tamed, when mutual and mature dependency is accepted as a realistic component of a gratifying human relationship, and when a harsh superego is replaced with an ego governed by the dictates of reality, the cardiac personality is ready to terminate psychotherapy because he or she is ready to love.

One of Sigmund Freud's (1914) most astute observations was that an individual who does not love is bound to fall ill. Anybody who has been involved with psychotherapy, either as a patient or therapist, learns the truth in Freud's remark.

As we help cardiac personalities face their inner and interpersonal worlds and offer them the humane, therapeutic relationship that we have described in the foregoing pages, we provide them with a corrective emotional experience. The experience we offer is one which our patients did not receive in growing up—a nurturing relationship which places their conflicts, their maturational needs, and their aches and pains in the forefront while ours are in the background.

One of the greatest benefits of a therapeutic relationship is that the patient learns how to love. Having been loved and understood consistently by the therapist over an extended period of time, the patient gradually identifies with the therapist and gives to others some of what he or she has received—love and understanding.

When patients have received the kind of therapy we have been discussing, they recognize that hatred is really an unpleasant emotion to feel, rarely serves constructive ends, and often leads to psychosomatic disturbances such as heart disease.

It is the thesis of this text that if the cardiac personality learns to love on a consistent basis and develops the capacity to enjoy intimacy and mutuality, he or she can prevent heart disease and/or reverse it. The title of the popular song "You've Got to Have Heart" implies that one has to love in order to live well, and that if one lives well, the heart will do its work well.

As I continue to work with more cardiac personalities, I now tell them early in treatment that when they can feel consistently loving, their heart disease and/or other problems will be substantially diminished. To accomplish this, they must confront their internal enemies—omnipotence, hostility, fear of dependency, and their corrupt and harsh superego.

Many therapists, and others, have asked me over the years what criteria I use when I am ready to say to a patient, "You are ready to try it on your own." With the aid of patients, counsel from colleagues, and wisdom from mentors and the literature (for example, Erikson 1950, Fine 1982, Freud 1914), I have finally arrived at having an image of the mentally healthy person. I use this image in diagnostically assessing my patients and have found it helpful in evaluating their progress in therapy.

First and foremost, mentally healthy people are able to love most of the time and in most relationships. When they feel or express hatred, they know it is a sign that they are experiencing feelings of vulnerability and they try to find out what they feel vulnerable about. In contrast to neurotic individuals who use hatred to protect themselves against feeling vulnerable, emotionally healthy men and women can acknowledge and accept limitations in themselves and others.

To enjoy a maximum of pleasure and a minimum of pain is also part of the healthy life. Cardiac personalities who have profited from psychotherapy recognize that real pleasure does not hurt themselves or others; otherwise, it is not healthy. Many cardiac personalities have indulged themselves in destructive and self-destructive pleasures such as telling some people off, submitting masochistically to others, eating too much fatty food, drinking too much liquor, and not exercising. Pleasure, to be healthy, enhances others and oneself over time. And, the healthiest and most constructive pleasure is participation in mutual love.

In reviewing the foregoing pages, we can observe that as our patients matured, they could experience a wider range of emotions and be able to empathize with a wider range of emotions in others. Implied throughout the preceding pages is the notion that mentally healthy people are not ashamed to feel sad, lonely, hurt, or angry. They are also free to laugh, cry, and feel excitement, joy, and even occasional bliss.

We are currently in the throes of a sexual revolution where sexual inhibitions are deemed neurotic and maladaptive by most mental health professionals and lay people. Therefore, part of being mature is enjoying a full and frequent sexual life.

Part of a mature sexual life is enjoying the pleasure that we give as well as the sexual satisfaction that we derive. Further, a healthy sexual life is one that combines lust with love. Love without excitement is not much fun; lust without tenderness is not very fulfilling.

One of the tremendous benefits which psychotherapy provides cardiac personalities is that when their omnipotent wishes are reduced, they can accept reality with more equanimity. When reality is accepted for what it is—sometimes beautiful and sometimes ugly—stress is always reduced to a minimum and, therefore, heart disease is held in check.

One of the greatest difficulties which cardiac personalities endure is not being able to accept the fact that life has its limitations, frustrations, and disappointments. They keep on trying to reach the paradise that's been lost or the Garden of Eden that's never been found. What is very difficult for them to face is that if they did not crave for so much, they would not be under so much stress. Much of the stress of cardiac personalities is caused by their inability to accept the fact that they will be rejected from time to time, occasionally treated unfairly even though they did not provoke it, and they will be hated even though they have behaved in a loving fashion.

Another task that is very challenging for cardiac personalities is learning how to overcome revenge. Many of them have been very emotionally abused by parents and others, and they want to place those who have hurt them in a similar position (A. Freud 1946). What we have learned from our patients is that when they feel or act revengefully, they are feeling like little children who are insisting on being loved by mature parents. They keep fighting the idea that their parents can't do better. Often, they turn their spouses, children, friends, and colleagues into parental figures and insist that these people compensate them for their horrible pasts. When their significant others don't indulge them, cardiac personalities do become bitter and revengeful. The therapeutically well-treated cardiac personality has learned in therapy that revenge is a self-destructive emotion and only hurts others and oneself.

When the cardiac personality (or any other individual) stops seeking revenge and accepts the past as something that "just had to be" (Erikson 1950), he or she is ready to participate in family life and give and take pleasure with all of its members. To enjoy a marriage or a parent-child relationship, the man or woman must stop living in the past. The marital partner is accepted and loved with his or her limitations and the same applies to other family members.

When the compulsiveness of work is understood and workaholism is relinquished, the patient begins to enjoy work. Hostility and competition have been diminished and achievements and accomplishments are not utilized to buttress unrecognized and unmastered vulnerabilities. Mentally healthy people, in contrast to their counterparts of yesteryear, do not regard work as punishment but as a means of fulfillment and gratification.

If cardiac personalities have been therapeutically helped, like all patients who have benefited from therapy, they can communicate well. Having been the recipients of empathetic communication, they begin to listen to others with more care and don't need to talk compulsively or finish other people's sentences for them. Communication becomes mutually pleasureful rather than as a tool to prove oneself or to lower a great deal of anxiety.

When the patient has accomplished this, he is close to what Reuben Fine (1982) has called *the analytic ideal*. As patients approach the analytic ideal and are essentially loving individuals, they get closer to another ideal—having a pure heart.

Epilogue: Straight from the Heart

Man is born broken.
He lives by mending.
— *Eugene O'Neill*

It has been stated frequently that every piece of writing, whether it is fiction or nonfiction, from the sciences or the arts, about psychotherapeutic matters or not, is an autobiography. This book is no exception.

Every patient who has been described and discussed in the foregoing pages is in one way or another the author. Any resemblance between him and the cardiac personalities whose dynamics and treatment have been portrayed is *not* coincidental! Furthermore, many of the theoretical concepts which have been presented here have been validated by my own personal experience with heart disease.

As of this writing, it is over 2 years since I suffered a

heart attack. These past 2 years have been the most painful, yet illuminating and constructive years of my life.

Facing the fact that I had a heart attack and suffer from heart disease was a severe blow to my omnipotence. For most of my life I had viewed myself as a healthy specimen who never was concerned about my mortality. After lying in a hospital bed in an intensive care unit for close to a week and told not to move, many of my omnipotent fantasies were shattered. Instead of utilizing most of my time working, reading, and writing, where I feel strong and competent, several hours of every day are now spent in exercise classes, stress management seminars, and in other arenas where I often feel like a vulnerable kindergartner. Instead of feeling like a "know-it-all," I have to accept that there's a lot I don't know and there may be many individuals who have a lot to teach me. This has been painful and not narcissistically gratifying!

Despite the fact that I was in personal analysis for many years and have done considerable self-analysis over the decades, my heart attack and subsequent involvement in the Dean Ornish Program at Beth Israel Hospital forced me to confront several unresolved neurotic issues in myself. I have also had to face the reappearance of old problems.

As I have actively participated in my support group, I have realized how much of a workaholic I am. I also became more aware of how much I craved admiration and affection. Of equal importance, it has become very clear to me that when the love and admiration I yearned for has not been forthcoming, I have been in a rage. Like the cardiac personalities in the foregoing pages, I needed much help in sensitizing myself to my powerful resentments. I also needed much help before I could acknowledge that I had deep dependency wishes which were and still are active.

I have found these past 2 years to be a most constructive time because I have been able to be freer of emotional conflict than in any other period of my life. I truly accept certain realities which I didn't and couldn't accept in the past. Now, whenever I start to feel anger toward someone or just fantasy it, I stop myself and say, "Let's see why you have to feel like a king. Let's see why you can't tolerate the hatred of someone who can't love you. What part of your personal history are you reliving?" I now believe my heart disease was caused mainly by the stress I was undergoing in my day-to-day life. I was very angry that I had not written a best seller. I was very angry that I hadn't cured every patient I treated. I was very angry that I didn't turn every student I taught into a genius. I was very angry that my wife, children, relatives, friends, and colleagues didn't always think I was the nicest guy they ever met.

Although I continue to exercise vigorously 6 days a week, do stress management daily, and am on a rigorous fat-free vegetarian diet, the decline in my heart disease (as demonstrated by all kinds of stress tests and other empirical observations) I am convinced is primarily due to my continuing to face my internal and interpersonal problems in my support group and with myself. When I'm sad, angry, or depressed, I start to converse with the little boy in myself. I start to recall how much I wanted to please my father who didn't talk to me for several days at a time if I didn't rank first in my class or hit a home run in a baseball game. I remind myself about my mother who told me frequently that girls are so much better than boys and that it was too bad I wasn't born a girl. These memories, I realize more than ever before, have shaped my view of current reality and made me more paranoid than I ever wanted to admit. They have a lot to do with my harsh superego and why I somaticized in exactly the same way my cardiac patients have done.

Because I genuinely accept as dynamics within myself my omnipotence, my hostility, my dependency yearnings, and my harsh superego, I can be more empathetic with my cardiac patients and with most of my other patients and students.

A statement from Harry Stack Sullivan which appears in all my writings seems truer today than it ever has: "We're all more human than otherwise."

References

Abend, S. (1989). Countertransference and psychoanalytic technique. *Psychoanalytic Quarterly* 58:374–395.

Abramov, L. (1976). Sexual life and sexual frigidity among women developing acute myocardial infarction. *Psychosomatic Medicine* 38:418–424.

Adler, K. (1967). Adler's individual psychology. In *Psychoanalytic Technique*, ed. B. Wolman. New York: Basic Books.

Alexander, F. (1939). Emotional factors in essential hypertension. *Psychosomatic Medicine* 1:173–180.

—— (1952). The psychosomatic approach in medicine. In *Dynamic Psychiatry*, ed. F. Alexander and H. Ross, pp. 369–400. Chicago: The University of Chicago Press.

—— (1965). *Psychosomatic Medicine: Its Principles and Application*. New York: W. W. Norton.

Alexander, F., and French, T. (1946). *Psychoanalytic Therapy*. New York: Ronald Press.

American Heart Association (1978). Diet and coronary heart disease. *Circulation* (pp. 762–766).

Angier, N. (1995). How biology affects behavior and vice versa. *The New York Times*, Science Section. May 30, 1995, p. 1.

Arieti, S. (1959). *American Handbook of Psychiatry*. New York: Basic Books.

Arlow, J. (1952). Anxiety patterns in angina pectoris. *Psychosomatic*

Medicine 14:461–469.

Ax, A. (1953). The physiological differentiation between fear and anger in humans. *Psychosomatic Medicine* 15:433–437.

Balint, M. (1948). *Primary Love and Psychoanalytic Technique.* London: Tavistock.

Benson, H. (1976). *The Relaxation Response.* New York: Avon Books.

———— (1977). Systemic hypertension and the relaxation response. *New England Journal of Medicine* 296:1152–1156.

———— (1984). *Beyond the Relaxation Response.* New York: Times Books.

———— (1987). *Your Maximum Mind.* New York: Times Books.

———— (1993). The relaxation response. In *Mind Body Medicine,* ed. D. Goleman and J. Gurin, pp. 233–258. Yonkers, NY *Consumers Union of United States.*

Bergler, E. (1969). *Selected Papers of Edmund Bergler.* New York: Grune & Stratton.

Blatt, S. (1995). Impact of perfectionism and need for approval on the brief treatment of depression. *Journal of Consulting and Clinical Psychology* 63:1:125–132.

Bliss, E., Rumel, W., and Branch, C. (1955). Psychiatric complication of mitral surgery: Report of death after electroshock therapy. *Archives of Neurology and Psychiatry* 74:249–261.

Bowlby, J. (1969, 1973, 1980). *Attachment and Loss* (3 vols.). New York: Basic Books.

Brenner, C. (1959). The masochistic character. *Journal of the American Psychoanalytic Association* 7:197–216.

Brody, J. (1995). Only vigorous exercise routine adds years to life. *New York Times,* April 19, 1995, p. 1.

Bruce, J. (1995). *Families in Focus.* New York: The Population Council.

Cameron, N. (1963). *Personality Development and Psychopathology: A Dynamic Approach.* Boston: Houghton Mifflin Company.

Cannon, W. (1929). *Bodily Changes in Pain, Hunger, Fear, and Rage. An Account of Recent Researches into the Function of Emotional Excitement.* New York: Appleton.

———— (1939). *The Wisdom of the Body.* New York: W. W. Norton.

———— (1963). *Bodily Changes in Pain, Hunger, Fear, and Rage.*

New York: W. W. Norton.

Charash, B. (1991). *Heart Myths: Setting the Record Straight on Prevention, Diagnosis, and Treatment.* New York: Viking Penguin.

Chassegut-Smiegel, J. (1984). *Creativity and Perversion.* New York: W. W. Norton.

Chopra, D. (1993). *Ageless Body, Timeless Mind.* New York: Harmony Books.

Coles, R. (1975). The cold, tough world of the affluent family. *Psychology Today,* November.

Consumer Reports on Health (1992). Heart attacks most likely to occur at dawn. Yonkers, NY, August.

Cortis, B. (1995). *Heart and Soul.* New York: Villard Books.

Cousins, N. (1976). Anatomy of an illness. *New England Journal of Medicine* 295:1458–1463.

―――― (1983). *The Healing Heart.* New York: W. W. Norton.

―――― (1989). *Head First: The Biology of Hope.* New York: Dutton.

Cutler, J., MacMahon, S., and Furberg, C. (1989). Controlled clinical trials of drug treatment for hypertension. *Hypertension* 13 (supplement 1):1–36—1–44.

Deutsch, H. (1965). *Neuroses and Character Types: Clinical Psychoanalytic Studies.* New York: International Universities Press.

Dunbar, F. (1943). *Psychosomatic Diagnosis.* New York: Paul B. Hoeber.

―――― (1944). Psychosomatic medicine. In *Psychoanalysis Today,* ed. S. Lorand, pp. 23–41. New York: International Universities Press.

―――― (1947). *Mind and Body: Psychosomatic Medicine.* New York: Random House.

Engel, G. (1950). *Physiological and Psychological Considerations.* Springfield, IL: Charles C Thomas.

―――― (1962). Anxiety and depression withdrawal: The primary affects of unpleasure. *International Journal of Psycho-Analysis* 43:89–97.

―――― (1967). The concept of psychosomatic disorder. *Journal of Psychosomatic Research* 11:3–10.

English, O., and Pearson, G. (1945). *Emotional Problems of Living.* New York: W.W. Norton.

Erikson, E. (1950). *Childhood and Society.* New York: W. W. Norton.

Eysenck, H. (1991). *Smoking, Personality and Stress: Psychosocial Factors in the Prevention of Cancer and Coronary Heart Disease.* New York: Springer-Verlag.

FDA Consumer Report (1994). The standard stress treadmill test falsely predicts heart disease. (November, p. 9) Yonkers, NY.

Fenichel, O. (1945). *The Psychoanalytic Theory of Neurosis.* New York: W. W. Norton.

Fine, R. (1982). *The Healing of the Mind* (2nd ed.). New York: The Free Press.

_____ (1988). *Troubled Men: The Psychology, Emotional Conflicts and Therapy of Men.* New York: Jossey Bass.

_____ (1990). *Love and Work.* New York: Continuum.

Flannery, R. (1990). *Becoming Stress-Resistant.* New York: Continuum.

Fox, H., Rizzo, N., and Gifford, S. (1954). Psychological observations of patients undergoing mitral surgery: A study of stress. *Psychosomatic Medicine* 16:186–195.

Freedman, A., Kaplan, H., and Sadock, B. (1976). *Modern Synopsis of Psychiatry* (2nd ed.). Baltimore: The Williams and Wilkins Company.

Freud, A. (1946). *The Ego and the Mechanisms of Defense.* New York: International Universities Press.

Freud, S. (1896). Further remarks on the neuropsychoses of defense. *Standard Edition* 3:159–185.

_____ (1897). Abstracts of the scientific writings of Dr. Sigmund Freud, 1887–1897. *Standard Edition (vol. 3).*

_____ (1905a). Three essays on the theory of sexuality. *Standard Edition* 7:125–243.

_____ (1905b). Jokes and their relation to the unconscious. *Standard Edition (vol. 8).*

_____ (1914). On narcissism. *Standard Edition* 14:67–102.

_____ (1923). The ego and the id. *Standard Edition* 19:1–66.

Friedman, M., and Rosenman, R. (1981). *Type A Behavior and Your Heart.* New York: Fawcett, Crest.

_____ (1984). *Treating Type A Behavior and Your Heart.* New York: Knopf.

Friedman, R., and Downey, J. (1995). Biology and the oedipus complex. *Psychoanalytic Quarterly* 64:234–264.

Funkenstein, D., King, S., and Drolette, M. (1953). The experimental evocation of stress. In *Symposium on Stress Army Medical Service Graduate School,* pp. 304–319. Washington, D.C.

Gardell, B., and Johansson, B. (1981). *Working Life: A Social Science Contribution to Work Reform.* New York: Wiley.

Gay, P. (1988). *Freud: A Life for Our Time.* New York: W. W. Norton.

Glick, P. (1977). Individualism, society, and social work. *Social Casework* Vol. 56, No. 10, pp. 37–46.

Glover, E. (1949). *Psychoanalysis: A Handbook for Medical Practitioners and Comparative Psychology* (2nd ed.). New York: Staples Press.

_____ (1960). *The Roots of Crime.* New York: International Universities Press.

Goleman, D., and Gurin, J. (1993). *Mind Body Medicine.* Yonkers, NY: Consumers Union of United States, Inc.

Grinker, R., and Robbins, F. (1954). *Psychosomatic Case Book.* New York: The Blakiston Company.

Grollman, A. (1929). Effect of psychic disturbance on cardiac output, blood pressure, and oxygen consumption. *American Journal of Physiology* 89:584–590.

Grossarth-Maticek, R., and Eysenck, H. (1990). Prophylactic effects of psychoanalysis on cancer-prone and coronary heart disease-prone probands as compared with control groups and behavior therapy groups. *Journal of Behavioral Therapy and Experimental Psychiatry* 21:91–99.

Hendin, H. (1975). *The Age of Sensation.* New York: W. W. Norton.

Hickam, J., Cargill, W., and Golden, A. (1948). Cardiovascular reaction to emotional stimuli: Effect on cardiac output, arteriovenous oxygen difference, arterial pressure, and peripheral resistance. *Journal of Clinical Investigation* 27:290–311.

Hollis, F. (1972). *Casework: A Psychosocial Therapy.* 2nd ed. New York: Random House.

House, J., Landis, K., and Umberson, D. (1988). Social relationships and health. *Science* 241:540–544.

Jacobs, T. (1986). On countertransference enactments. *Journal of the American Psychoanalytic Association* 43:289–307.

Jacobson, E. (1971). *Depression: Comparative Studies of Normal, Neurotic, and Psychotic Conditions.* Madison, CT: International Universities Press.

Jones, E. (1953). *The Life and Work of Sigmund Freud: The Formative*

Years and the Great Discoveries (vol. 1). New York: Basic Books.

Kadushin, A. (1972). *The Social Work Interview*. New York: Columbia University Press.

Kaplan, J., Manuck, S., and Clarkson, T. (1982). Social status, environment, and atherosclerosis in cynomolgus monkeys. *Arteriosclerosis* 2(5):359–368.

Kaplan, N. (1987). Misdiagnosis of systemic hypertension and recommendations for improvement. *American Journal of Cardiology* 60:1383–1385.

Kaplan, S. (1956). Psychological aspects of cardiac disease: A study of patients experiencing mitral commissurotomy. *Psychosomatic Medicine* 18:221–231.

Kardiner, A. (1945). *The Psychological Frontiers of Society*. New York: Columbia University Press.

Kelman, H., and Vollmerhausen, J. (1967). On Horney's psychoanalytic techniques. Developments and perspectives. In *Psychoanalytic Techniques,* ed. B. Wolman. New York: Basic Books.

Kernberg, O. (1967). Borderline personality organization. *Journal of the American Psychoanalytic Association* 15:641–685.

———— (1988). Clinical dimensions of masochism. *Journal of the American Psychoanalytic Association* 36:1005–1029.

———— (1995). *Love Relations: Normality and Pathology*. New Haven, CT: Yale University Press.

Klein, M. (1932). *The Psychoanalysis of Children*. London: Hogarth Press.

Kohut, H. (1977). *The Restoration of the Self*. New York: International Universities Press.

Krugman, S. (1991). Male vulnerability and the transformation of shame. In *On Men: Redefining Roles,* ed. W.S. Pollack. Cambridge, MA: The Cambridge Series, The Cambridge Hospital, Harvard Medical School.

Krystal, H. (1979). Alexithymia and psychotherapy. *Journal of Psychotherapy* 33:17–30.

Kunz, J., and Finkel, A. (1987). *The American Medical Association Family Guide*. New York: Random House.

Lacey, J., and Van Lehn, R. (1952). Differential emphasis in somatic response to stress. *Psychosomatic Medicine* 14:71–77.

Langford, H. (1989). Nonpharmacological therapy of hypertension.

Commentary on diet and blood pressure. *Hypertension* 13:98–102.

Langley, R., and Levy, R. (1977). *Wife Beating: The Silent Crisis.* New York: Dutton.

Lasch, C. (1978). *The Culture of Narcissism.* New York: W. W. Norton.

Lazare, A. (1987). Shame and humiliation in the medical encounter. *Archives of Internal Medicine* 147:1653–1658.

Lazarus, R., and Folkman, S. (1984). *Stress, Appraisal, and Coping.* New York: Springer.

Lerner, J., and Noy, P. (1968). Somatic complaints in psychiatric disorders: Social and cultural factors. *International Journal of Social Psychiatry* 14:145–150.

Levant, R. (1995). *Masculinity Reconstructed: Changing the Rules of Manhood at Work, in Relationships, and in Family Life.* New York: Dutton.

Lidz, T. (1959). General concepts of psychosomatic medicine. In *American Handbook of Psychiatry,* ed. S. Arieti. New York: Basic Books.

Lindermann, E. (1941). Observations on psychiatric sequellae to surgical operations in women. *American Journal of Psychiatry* 98:132–139.

Lowen, A. (1988). *Love, Sex, and your Heart. The Health-Happiness Connection.* New York: Penguin Books.

Lutz, W. (1964). Marital incompatibility. In *Social Work and Social Problems,* ed. N. Cohen. New York: National Association of Social Workers.

Lynch, J. (1977). *The Broken Heart: The Medical Consequences of Loneliness.* New York: Basic Books.

_____ (1985). *The Language of the Heart: The Human Body in Dialogue.* New York: Basic Books.

Mahler, M. (1966). Notes on the development of basic moods: The depressive affect in psychoanalysis. In *Psychoanalysis—A General Psychology,* ed. R. Lowenstein, L. Newman, M. Schur and A. Solnit, pp. 152–168. New York: International Universities Press.

May, M. (1991). Observations on countertransference, addiction, and treatability. In *Psychoanalytic Approaches to Addiction,* ed. A. Smaldino. New York: Brunner/Mazel.

May, R. (1969). *Love and Will.* New York: W. W. Norton.

McDougall, J. (1985). *Theatre of the Mind: Illusion and Truth on the Psychoanalytic Stage*. New York: Basic Books.

_____ (1989). *Theatres of the Body*. New York: W. W. Norton.

Menninger, K. (1934). Polysurgery and polysurgic addiction. *Psychoanalytic Quarterly* 3:173–199.

The Menninger Letter (April 1995). Low cholesterol level can lead to depression, p. 4.

Moore, B., and Fine, B. (1990). *Psychoanalytic Terms and Concepts*. New Haven, CT: Yale University Press.

Moore, T. (1995). *Deadly Medicine*. New York: Simon and Schuster.

Moses-Hrushovski, R. (1994). *Hiding Behind Power Struggles as a Character Defense*. Northvale, NJ: Jason Aronson.

Nee, L. (1995). Effects of psychosocial interactions at a cellular level. *Social Work* 40(2): 259–262.

Nemiah, J. (1978). Alexithymia and psychosomatic illness. *Journal of Continuing Education in Psychiatry*, pp. 25–37.

Nicholson, A. (Spring 1995). The Ornish program: How are they doing five years later? *Good Medicine*, pp.18–19.

Novick, J., and Novick, K. (1991). Some comments on masochism and the delusion of omnipotence from a developmental perspective. *Journal of the American Psychoanalytic Association* 39:307–332.

Offit, A. (1995). *The Sexual Self: How Character Shapes Sexual Experience*. Northvale, NJ: Jason Aronson.

Ornish, D. (1990). *Reversing Heart Disease*. New York: Ballantine Books.

Palmare, E. (1969). Predicting longevity. *Gerontology*, Winter issue.

Parens, H., and Saul, L. (1971). *Dependence in Man*. New York: International Universities Press.

Patlak, M. (1994). Women and heart disease. *FDA Consumer*, November, 7:7–10.

Pelletier, K. (1992). *Mind as Healer, Mind as Slayer. (revised ed.)* New York: Delacorte.

_____ (1993). Between mind and body: Stress, emotions and health. In *Mind Body Medicine*, ed. D. Goleman and J. Gurin, pp. 19–38, Yonkers, NY: Consumers Union of United States, Inc.

Perry, H. (1982). *Psychiatrist of America. The Life of Harry Stack Sullivan*. Cambridge, MA: Harvard University Press.

Poland, W. (1994). The gift of laughter: On the development of a sense of humor in clinical analysis. In *The Use of Humor in Psychotherapy*, ed. H. Strean. Northvale, NJ: Jason Aronson.

Priest, W., Zaks, M., Yacorzynski, G., and Boshes, B. (1957). The neurologic, psychiatric, and psychological aspects of cardiac surgery. *Medical Clinician of North America* 41:155–162.

Rahe, R. (1975). Epidemiological studies of life change and illness. *International Journal of Psychiatry in Medicine* Vol. 6, Nos. 1 & 2, pp. 133–146.

Reich, W. (1949). *Character Analysis* (3rd ed.). New York: Orgone Institute Press.

Reik, T. (1941). *Masochism in Modern Man*. New York: Grove Press.

Reiser, M. (1966). Toward an integrated psychoanalytic and physiologic theory of psychosomatic disorders. In *Psychoanalysis—A General Psychology*, ed. R. Lowenstein, D. Newman, M. Schur, and A. Solnit, pp. 570–582. New York: International Universities Press.

Reiser, M., and Bakst, H. (1959). Psychology of cardiovascular disorders. In *American Handbook of Psychiatry*, ed. M. Reiser and H. Bakst. New York: Basic Books.

Reiser, M., Reeves, R., and Armington, J. (1955). The effect of variations in laboratory procedure and experimenter upon the bassis tocardiogram, heart rate, and blood pressure of healthy young men. *Psychosomatic Medicine* 17:185–191.

Renik, O. (1993). Analytic interaction: Conceptualizing technique in light of the analyst's irreducible subjectivity. *Psychoanalytic Quarterly* 62:553–571.

Rensch, J. (1948). The infantile personality: The core problem of psychosomatic medicine. *Psychosomatic Medicine* 10:137–151.

Rogers, C. (1951). *Client-centered therapy*. Boston: Houghton Mifflin.

Rossman, M. (1993). Imagery: Learning to use the mind's eye. In *Mind Body Medicine*, ed. D. Goleman and J. Gurin, pp. 291–300. Yonkers, NY: Consumers Union of United States, Inc.

Sacks, M. (1993). Exercise for stress control. In *Mind Body Medicine*, ed. D.Goleman and J. Gurin, pp. 315–327. Yonkers, NY: Consumers Union of United States, Inc.

Sacks, O. (1995). *An Anthropologist on Mars: Seven Paradoxical*

Tales. New York: Alfred A. Knopf.

Saul, L. (1976). *The Psychodynamics of Hostility.* Northvale, NJ: Jason Aronson.

Schacter, J. (1957). Pain, fear, and anger in hypertensives and normotensives: A psychophysiological study. *Psychosomatic Medicine* 19:17–21.

Schafer, R. (1983). *The Analytic Attitude.* New York: Basic Books.

———— (1995). Aloneness in the countertransference. *Psychoanalytic Quarterly* 64:3:496–516.

Schardt, D. (1995). For men only. *Nutrition Action Newsletter 22 (no.5):4–5.* Washington, DC: Center for Science in the Public Interest.

Scherwitz, L., Berton, K., and Leventhal, H. (1978). Type A behavior, self-involvement and cardiovascular response. *Psychosomatic Medicine* 40(8):593–609.

Schneider, D. (1967). *Psychoanalysis of Heart Attack.* Easthampton, NY: The Alexa Press.

Schur, M. (1951). Basic problems of psychosomatic medicine. In *A Handbook of Psychoanalysis,* ed. H. Herma and G. Kurth, pp. 237–266. Cleveland, OH: The World Publishing Company.

Selye, H. (1950). *The Physiology and Pathology of Exposure to Stress: A Treatise Based on the Concepts of the General-Adaptation-Syndrome and the Diseases of Adaptation.* Montreal: Acta, Inc.

———— (1978). *The Stress of Life.* (2nd ed) New York: McGraw Hill.

Selye, H., and Heuser, G. (1955). *Fifth Annual Report on Stress.* New York: Medical Publications.

Sheridan, M., and Kline, K. (1984). Psychogenic and psychophysiologic disorders. In *Adult Psychopathology: A Social Work Perspective.* New York: The Free Press.

Sifneos, P. (1967). *Clinical Observations on Some Patients Suffering From a Variety of Psychosomatic Diseases. Proceedings of the Seventh European Conference on Psychosomatic Research.* Basel, Switzerland: Kargel.

Sigerist, H. (1951). *A History of Medicine.* New York: Oxford University Press.

Singer, M. (1977). Psychological dimensions in psychosomatic patients.

Psychotherapy and Psychosomatic Medicine 28:13–27.

Slakter, E. (1987). *Countertransference*. Northvale, NJ: Jason Aronson.

Sperling, M. (1949). The role of the mother in psychosomatic disorders in children. *Psychosomatic Medicine* 11:377–385.

———— (1950). Mucous colitis associated with phobias. *Psychoanalytic Quarterly* 3:318–326.

———— (1952). Psychotherapeutic techniques in psychosomatic medicine. In *Specialized Techniques in Psychotherapy,* ed. G. Bychowski and J.L. Despert, pp. 279–302. New York: Grove Press.

Stearns, P., and Stearns, C. (1986). *Anger: The Struggle for Emotional Control in America's History.* Chicago: University of Chicago Press.

Sternschein, I. (1975). Psychosomatic disorders. In *Personality Development and Deviation,* ed. G. Wiedeman. New York: International Universities Press.

Strean, H. (1970). The use of the patient as consultant. In *New Approaches in Child Guidance,* ed. H. Strean. Metuchen, NJ: Scarecrow Press.

———— (1980). *The Extramarital Affair.* New York: The Free Press.

———— (1985). *Resolving Marital Conflicts.* New York: John Wiley and Sons.

———— (1990). *Resolving Resistances in Psychotherapy.* New York: Brunner/Mazel.

———— (1993a). *Resolving Counterresistances in Psychotherapy.* New York: Brunner/Mazel.

———— (1993b). *Jokes: Their Meaning and Purpose.* Northvale, NJ: Jason Aronson.

———— (1994a). *Essentials of Psychoanalysis.* New York: Brunner/Mazel.

———— (1994b). *Therapists Who Have Sex with their Patients.* New York: Brunner/Mazel.

———— (1995a). *Psychotherapy with the Unattached.* Northvale, NJ: Jason Aronson.

———— (1995b). Countertransference and theoretical predilections as observed in some psychoanalytic candidates. *Canadian Journal of Psychoanalysis* 3:1:105–124.

Sullivan, H.S. (1953). *The Interpersonal Theory of Psychiatry.* New York: W. W. Norton.

Sussman, M. (1992). *A Curious Calling: Unconscious Motivations for Practicing Psychotherapy.* Northvale, NJ: Jason Aronson.

U.S. Department of Health and Human Services (1988). National Institute of Health Publication No. 88–2724. May.

Von Bertalanffy, L. (1964). The mind–body problem—a new view. *Psychosomatic Medicine* 26:29–45.

Waelder, R. (1941). The scientific approach to casework with special emphasis on psychoanalysis. In *Principles and Techniques in Social Casework*, ed. C. Kasius. New York: Family Service Association of America.

Wahrer, A., and Burchell, R. (1980). Male sexual dysfunction associated with coronary heart disease. *Archives of Sexual Behavior* 9:69–75.

Walker, C. (1995). *Long Time Coming: A Black Athlete's Coming-of-age in America.* New York: Grove Press.

Weiss, R. (1990). *Staying the Course: The Emotional and Social Lives of Men Who Do Well at Work.* New York: Fawcett Colombine.

Wiedeman, G. (1975). *Personality Development and Deviation.* New York: International Universities Press.

Williams, R. (1989). *The Trusting Heart.* New York: Times Books.

_____ (1993). Hostility and the heart. In *Mind Body Medicine,* ed. D. Goleman and J. Gurin, pp. 65–85. Yonkers, NY: Consumers Union of United States, Inc.

Wilson, E. (1978). *On Human Nature.* Cambridge, MA: Harvard University Press.

Winnicott, D. (1966). Psychosomatic illness in its positive and negative aspects. *International Journal of Psycho-Analysis* 47:510–516.

_____ (1971). *Therapeutic Consultations in Child Psychiatry.* New York: Basic Books.

The Winston Dictionary (1943). Philadelphia: The John C. Winston Company.

Wittkower, E. (1969). A global survey of psychosomatic medicine. *International Journal of Psychiatry* 7:499–524.

Wolff, S., and Goodell, H. (1962). *Behavior Science in Clinical Medicine.* Springfield, IL: Charles C Thomas.

Wolff, S., and Wolff, H. (1947). *Human Gastric Function: An Experimental Study of a Man and His Stomach.* (2nd ed.) New York: Oxford University Press.

Wolfin, H. (1950). *Life Stress and Bodily Disease.* Baltimore: The Williams and Wilkins Company.

Index

LIBRARY, UNIVERSITY COLLEGE CHESTER